The Survival Medicine Guide

Essential Skills for Life-Threatening Emergencies

Copyright © All rights reserved.

No part of this book may be reproduced, in any form or by any means, without permission in writing from the author or publisher, except for brief excerpts used in reviews

TABLE OF CONTENTS

TABLE OF CONTENTS 3

DISCLAIMER 7

HEALTH AND WELLNESS: WHAT IS HEALTH? 8

    Physical Examination 9

    10 Medical Supplies You Need to Have in Your House 10

    An Ingenious Way to Stockpile Prescription Medicines 12

    Medicines that Are Safe to Take After Their Expiration Date 14

    The Biggest Mistakes You Can Make in a Blackout 16

    The Only 4 Antibiotics People Should Stockpile 18

MENTAL HEALTH 20

    1. STRESS 20

        What Symptoms Can Intense Stress Cause? 21

    2. DEPRESSION 21

        Symptoms and Signs 21

SKIN AND SKIN APPENDAGES 22

    1. CORNS 24

    2. WARTS 25

    3. INSECT BITES AND STINGS 25

        When Should I Worry? 26

        Warning Signs 26

        How Can I Be Prepared? 26

    4. NAIL TRAUMA 27

        What Can I Do at Home? 27

        Ingrown Toenails (Onychocryptosis) 27

        Dealing Effectively with Ingrown Nails Without Leaving Home 27

HEAD AND NECK 30

    1. Headaches and Muscle Contractures 30

        Types of Headaches 30

        Treatment Options 33

- 2. Neck Pain 34
  - Treatment 34
  - When Should I Worry? 35
- 3. Eyes and Appendages of the Eye 36
  - Red Eye 36
  - Cataracts 39
  - Eye Pain 41
  - Stye 42
  - Blepharitis 43

RESPIRATORY SYSTEM 44

- 1. Cough 45
  - Most Common Causes 45
  - Treatment 46
  - When Should I Worry? 47
  - What Does Expectoration Mean? 47
- 2. Ear, Nose, and Throat 47
  - Ear 48
  - Nose 52
  - Throat 54
- 3. Airway Obstruction 56
  - What Can I Do if I Am Alone? 57
  - Tracheotomy: A Life-Saving Procedure When Help Is Not Available 57

GASTROINTESTINAL SYSTEM 59

- 1. Mouth Problems 59
  - Cold Sores 59
  - Thrush 59
  - Canker Sores 60
  - Papillitis (Lie Bumps) 61
- 2. Teeth Problems 61
  - Toothache and Gingivitis 61
  - Dental Trauma 62
  - Dental Abscess 62
- 3. Vomiting and Diarrhea (Stomach Flu) 64
  - Symptoms 65
  - Treatment 65

UROGENITAL SYSTEM 66
1. Urinary Urgency and Urge Incontinence 67
Common Causes of Urinary Urgency and Urge Incontinence 68
Straining to Urinate 76

MUSCULOSKELETAL SYSTEM 82
1. Osteoporosis 83
2. Arthritis 84
Rheumatoid Arthritis 84
Osteoarthritis 85
Gout 86
3. Muscle Pain (Myalgia) 88
Muscle Hematoma 88
Muscle Abscess 89
4. Sprain 90
Diagnosis 91
Treatment 92
5. Fractures 92

CARDIOVASCULAR SYSTEM 95
1. High Blood Pressure 103
Treatment 105
Preventing Hypertension and Keeping Blood Pressure Low 107
2. Cardiovascular Emergencies 108
Chest Pain 108

ENDOCRINE SYSTEM 109
1. Pancreas: Diabetes Mellitus Types 1 and 2 112
Pancreatitis 113
Diabetes Mellitus (DM) 116
2. Obesity and Metabolic Syndrome 118
Nutritional Supplements in the Bariatric Patient 120

NERVOUS SYSTEM 121
1. Stroke 123
Symptoms 124
2. Seizures 125
How Do I Know Someone Is Having a Seizure and What Should I Do? 125

IMMUNE SYSTEM 126

1. What Can Disturb My Immune System?	127
2. How Do I Strengthen My Immune System?	127

A FEW RECIPES PUT TOGETHER FOR YOU 129
1. A Natural DIY Antibiotic Salve Recipe to Keep Around 129
2. A Simple "At-Home" Protocol for the Flu and Other Respiratory Issues 131
3. How to Make Calcium Pills from Eggshells 135

PLANTS WITH MEDICINAL PROPERTIES 138
1. Painkillers 138
2. Antibiotics 140
3. Anti-Inflammatories 142

DISCLAIMER

This book is not a medical guide and should not be used as such.

This information is made available with the knowledge that the publisher, editor, and authors do not offer any legal or medical advice. In case you are ill you should always consult with your primary care physician or another medical specialist.

This book does not claim to contain and indeed does not contain all the information available on the subject of home remedies.

While the authors, editor, and publisher have gone to great lengths to provide the most useful and accurate collection of knowledge about home remedies, there may still exist typographical and/or content errors.

This book was created so that people can read it and learn from it, in case of an extraordinary event like an Apocalypse that changes the World as we know it, leading to the collapse of the states, society, medical system, law and order AND the dissolution of the social fabric. In this regard, this book's purpose is to save some of the knowledge that will be lost in this wide spread collapse. It is not meant to treat or cure anyone! Do not use this book for this purpose!

The authors, editor, and publisher shall incur no liability or be held responsible to any person or entity regarding any loss of life or injury, alleged or otherwise, that happened directly or indirectly as a resultof using the information contained in this book. It is your own responsibility and if you want to use one of the many remedies or anything else from this book you should always consult with your physician first.

Some of the home remedies found within this book do not comply with FDA guidelines.

The information in the book has not been reviewed, tested or approved by any official testing body or government agency.

The authors and editor of this book make no guarantees of any kind, expressed or implied, regarding the final results obtained by applying the information found in this book. Taking any of the medicines and using any of the methods described in the book will be done at your own risk.

The authors, editor, and publisher hold no responsibility for the misuse of a remedy or drug using the contents of this book, or any and all consequences to your health or that of others that may result.

Some names and identifying details have been changed to protect the privacy of the authors and other individuals.

By reading past this point you hereby agree to be bound by this disclaimer, or you may return this book within the guarantee time period for a full refund.

HEALTH AND WELLNESS: WHAT IS HEALTH?

According to the World Health Organization (WHO), health is defined as a state of complete physical, mental, and social well-being and not merely the absence of disease or infirmity.

This concept is important because it embraces psychological and social well-being, which is not present in other definitions. Therefore, we understand that mental health is an element to be taken into account. As for physical health itself, the concept, which is understood by almost everyone, refers to the absence of visible disease.

Through the general physical examination, we can make diagnostic approaches. Semiological evaluation is an assessment we should all be aware of since it is an important tool to establish the diagnosis as the first step in the approach to the disease.

A proper evaluation begins with an interview to find out the medical history of the affected person and when the present illness began. It is important to take into account whether the person is allergic to any medication or component in case drugs are administered later. The physical exam is a simple evaluation of the entire body.

It is important to be systematic, which means to have a methodical evaluation so nothing is left behind and forgotten. Remember to pay special attention to the part of the body where the patient refers to the symptoms, and focus on that area.

Below is an example of a current illness interrogation and a simple way to perform the physical examination in an orderly and efficient way.

PAST	<ul><li>Cancer or chronic illness in the family</li><li>Medical and surgical history</li><li>Allergic reactions (to food or drugs). What kind of reaction? Did you need hospitalization?</li><li>Use of medication</li><li>What kind of work do you do?</li><li>Sleeping hours</li><li>Physical activity</li></ul>
PRESENT	<ul><li>When and how did the symptoms start? Do you associate them with anything in particular?</li><li>Have you ever had these symptoms before?</li><li>Are you taking any medication to improve? Which one? How many times a day? Does it work?</li></ul>

In the case of specific pains, I like the patient to point out exactly where the pain is, and I ask them to do so with only one finger. That way I can make sure they point out the place where they have the most pain rather than scattering it.

The questions in the table are general, and it is important to delve as deeply as necessary into the patient's main symptom in order to take a diagnostic approach. When you can't ask for specialized help, interrogation is the main tool available. Therefore, it is necessary to use all the time that is required to orientate yourself.

If the patient is a child or an elderly person with dementia, the history is taken with the help of a family member or from what you yourself have witnessed. Try to remember important information, such as recent falls or a decrease in normal activities.

It is also important to know the person's recent contacts if an infectious disease is suspected. Currently, with the issue of the COVID-19 pandemic, this is one of the most important questions since it is a disease with a high rate of contagion. Remember that the therapy to be applied will be based on the diagnosis; therefore, we must be as precise as possible.

Physical Examination

In the physical examination, we must go from the biggest to the most specific. The observation of the face and the position that the person adopts can take us closer to the diagnosis.

If the patient has pained face or *facies dolorosa* or if he or she is held in a position that looks uncomfortable or out of the ordinary to relieve the pain, this is an antalgic position.

Thus, when a patient complains of pain, for example, we first check his vital signs (heart rate, number of breaths per minute), and from there, we continue to palpate.

When the patient cannot adequately express the intensity of the pain, a scale of numbers from 1 to 10 is used, where 1 is the lowest and 10 is the highest. If the patient cannot speak and has problems communicating, there is also the scale with facial expressions. Both are shown below.

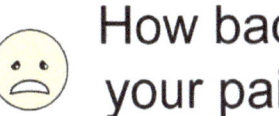 How bad is your pain?

1: Huh, I guess it's there...
2: It's mildly distracting
3: I can usually ignore it
4: It's there, but I can do stuff
5: It interferes with some things
6: It disrupts daily life
7: I can barely do anything
8: It's hard to talk & listen
9: I can barely move
10: I am bedridden. Help!

MissLunaRose12, Own work, CC BY-SA 4.0

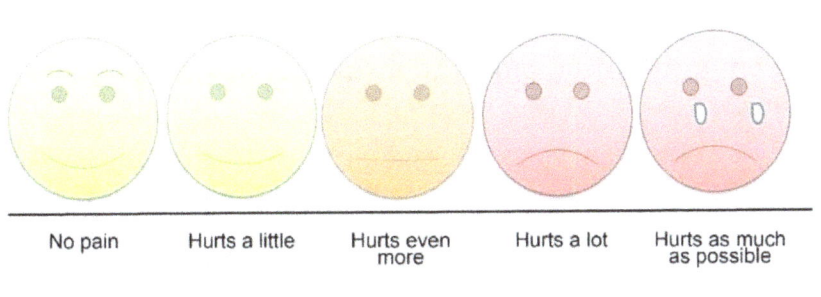

Robert Weis, Own work, CC BY-SA 4.0

To make the physical evaluation more comfortable for the patient, try to get to the site of the discomfort by the end of the exam.

If his or her left leg is painful, examine the entire body before reaching that leg. This helps the person to be relaxed and confident that you will not hurt them or cause pain.

For those who are traumatized, always remember to examine the patient from the front and the back. When I did my surgery residency, I remember being on call when I received an emergency call about a decompensated patient who had a gunshot wound that appeared to have caused no damage beyond a burn on the skin. However, the patient had been in the emergency room for 24 hours and was getting worse.

When I arrived, the patient was in bad condition, with a very high heart rate and in a lot of pain. WhenI turned the patient over, he had another wound on his back that no one had noticed. That wound had penetrated the abdominal cavity, and the patient had to undergo emergency surgery.

Sometimes amid the stress of being in front of one or more injured people, we can inadvertently skip some parts of the physical examination. That's why we have to be methodical. You can start the evaluation at the head and finish at the feet without leaving anything out.

Find your method and practice it.

10 Medical Supplies You Need to Have in Your House

As times change, we must change alongside it. If the year 2020 has taught us anything, it is that life itself is fragile and good health is underrated. We really never know what is going to happen and so there is a need for us to be prepared. March 2020 left the entire world standing in utter surprise and confusion as the COVID 19 spread like wild fire throughout countries and continents. The world was thrown into a state of chaos, not knowing the adequate reaction to such a deadly pandemic. Lives were lost from the disease, hunger, other health issues, and lack of access to the health centers and medications. In 2020 it was the pandemic, but it could be any disaster such as an earthquake, a tsunami, or an economic crisis. Therefore, we must have certain medical supplies at home that are useful in the event of an emergency.

Having the right medical supplies ranging from medical equipment to medications is key to surviving any medical emergency in the face of a disaster.

Naproxen is a medication that belongs to the NSAID (Non-Steroidal Anti-inflammatory Drug) family.It is very effective in treating moderate pain, swelling, and even in cases of a fever. It has proven to be very effective in relieving pain caused by osteoarthritis, rheumatoid arthritis, bursitis, gout attacks, muscles pains, headaches, sprains, menstrual cramps, and dental pains. Naproxen generates rapid and long lasting relief. Definitely a necessity at home.

Loratadine is also a fundamental supply in homes, useful in cases of allergies such as allergic rhinitis (hay fever) and urticaria (allergic skin rash). It is effective in the relief of pruritus, watery eyes, runny nose, and sneezing associated with seasonal allergies or flu. It is a second generation antihistaminic medication which can be used both in older people and children above the age of 2.

Having a **thermometer** at home makes it easy to determine body temperature. A thermometer measures the temperature of the body and tells us if a person has a normal temperature, a fever (temperature above 38 degrees Celsius) or a low temperature (less than 35 degrees Celsius). This comes in very handy in pediatric emergencies. Fever is frequent in kids and they frequently suffer convulsions from high temperature. Having a thermometer at home helps us know when to control body temperature and prevent convulsions or other complications of a fever.

Acetaminophen is the number one drug for fevers and headaches. It is a non-opioid analgesic (pain-relieving) and antipyretic (fever-treating) drug used for treatment of mild to moderate pain and fever. Acetaminophen can be administered to kids and adults alike as it comes in the form of pills, liquids, injections and rectal suppository. It has proven to be effective in treating flu like symptoms.

Gauze sponges come in handy in the home as good materials for cleaning wounds, dressing wounds and applying pressure on a bleeding surface of the body. Since they are sterile, they serve as a protective barrier between the injured part of the body and the external surface.

Bandages are very effective for treating and protecting minor injuries permitting a germ-free healing process. They are useful in cases such as small cuts, scratches etc. They have a protective function that allows the injured person to go about their daily activities without exposing the injury to infections.

Medical gloves should be a house hold item. In cases of injuries, bleeding, wound dressing and cleaning, you must wear gloves. As we all know, our hands carry a large number of germs as we go about our activities touching surfaces, objects or people; therefore the use of gloves to access injured parts of the body, remove foreign objects from an airway, etc. is very important.

Alcohol and alcohol swabs have become one of the most sold medical supplies in recent times as COVID 19 taught us the importance of disinfecting surfaces and objects. It is also a well-known fact that many people are prone to injuries such as minor cuts, burns or scrapes. In such cases, a little amount of alcohol or an alcohol swab is your best bet. Alcohol can be used to destroy germs that could be present in open wounds. Sniffing alcohol/alcohol swabs has demonstrated effectiveness in reducing nausea and vomiting too.

Oral rehydration solution (ORS) should be readily available in every home. There are many reasons why people may present with gastrointestinal upset leading to vomiting and diarrhea. In such cases there is loss of liquid and electrolytes causing the affected person to suffer dehydration which can in turn lead to shock. This is frequent in kids below the age of 5. Having ORS at home helps us prevent complications from diarrhea and vomiting by replacing lost liquid and electrolytes.

Omeprazole is the go-to medication for stomach upset, heart burns and other acid related issues. It works by blocking acid production in the cells of the stomach. Many people suffer from gastritis and ulcers and sometimes eating certain foods or overeating might cause stomach upset. In such cases omeprazole will be functional in eliminating the discomfort and bring relief.

The above mentioned medications are over the counter drugs that could be bought in stores or pharmacies without prescription, which makes them readily available for home use. However, it is always important to consult your physician before use. These supplies and medications are all very useful in emergencies and having them at home can help save lives and in other cases prevent health complications. Remember, that in the past year people have suffered losses that could have been prevented if they only had some or all of these medical supplies in their homes. Venezuela as we know is experiencing an economic crisis that has made foods and medical supplies very scarce. People have died due to the absence of these simple medical supplies in Venezuela. So yes, there is a very strong need for us to equip our homes with medical supplies and stay prepared.

An Ingenious Way to Stockpile Prescription Medicines

If you're like many Americans these days, it's likely that you have at least one medication that you need to take regularly. It is also likely that this medication is one that is essential, meaning that being without it may constitute an emergency. Things like insulin, inhalers, and blood pressure medications are part of daily life for millions of people; yet most of those people do not have a plan in place for what they'd do if the medication were suddenly unavailable.

In the wake of the COVID-19 pandemic, many are seeing that this scenario is becoming closer and closer to reality. Between the public scrambling to fill prescriptions out of fear for their health to pharmaceutical production being halted due to quarantines and shut downs, many medications became temporarily scarce. While pharmacies and pharmaceutical companies have done their best to mitigate the effects of various shortages, the situation highlighted for many that they would be in nearly immediate danger if their medication became suddenly and indefinitely unavailable.

Becoming suddenly unable to acquire necessary medication is certainly a frightening thought, but there are some ways in which you may be able to build a stash of emergency medication. It may take a while to stockpile a reasonable supply – prescription medications are relatively well-controlled, both by pharmacies and health insurance companies.

Some "easy" methods for stockpiling meds (like purchasing illegally online or skipping doses) should be avoided for safety reasons, but the following are a few ways to start building a stash of your medication safely and legally:

1.) Refill Your Prescriptions as Soon as Possible

It is standard practice to have prescriptions refilled a day or two before they run out, but most insurances will allow for refills to be filled and covered up to a week in advance of the current supply running out. The best way to find out when you can get a refill is to call your insurance directly, as medical providers typically don't know the ins and outs of insurance coverage. Building up a backup medication supply this way is slow but takes minimal effort. By refilling prescriptions three to five days before they run out you can put aside three to five days of medication for emergencies.

This method is slow, and if you want to have more of a supply for peace of mind you may also be able to get a full refill if you claim to have lost your medication. Most insurance companies only allow full replacement of a lost prescription once or twice a year, but even once is enough to have a full month worth of your medication for a stockpile. It can't hurt to ask at your pharmacy whether they are able to replace a lost prescription.

2.) Manage Symptoms Alternatively when Possible

This is not to say "stop taking your meds and try alternative treatments"; rather, it is just to say that many conditions requiring pharmaceutical management can also be greatly affected by lifestyle changes as well. Take insulin for example – while it is less the case for type 1 diabetics, both type 1 and type 2 diabetes can benefit from dietary changes and more physical activity. Consuming fewer sugars and processed carbohydrates can result in a more stable blood sugar, often requiring less insulin.

If you use insulin on a scale according to blood sugar readings, try making some lifestyle changes and you may see that you have more insulin left over at the end of each month. If this becomes the case, refill as soon as possible but continue using the existing supply before opening the refill. Try to keep the newest supply as your backup or stockpile supply, keeping in mind that expired insulin is better than nothing but may be less effective as time passes.

Managing conditions alternatively can also be useful in setting aside some medications for things like pain or heart conditions. With pain, many alternative therapies have been proven effective – things like ice, relaxation techniques, certain foods, and even music can curb the need for medication, allowing you to save as many doses as you'd like for a stockpile. Skipping doses of pain medication, unlike other medications, is not harmful and can even have a positive effect on pain tolerance in general. For things like blood pressure or heart rate, calming routines and managing stressors can result in less frequent need for medication. Doses of things like metoprolol or lisinopril should absolutely not be skipped without physician approval, but these medications are often used within parameters which means that if your heart rate or blood pressure is within an acceptable range, there is no need for the dose.

3.) Ask Your Doctor about Using Your Medication with Parameters

As previously mentioned, sometimes medications for heart rate and blood pressure are used with parameters. This is also the case with some insulin use, referred to as being on a "sliding scale". If you feel that your medication may be able to be used on an as-needed basis, ask your physician! Putting parameters on the use of a particular medication involves more work in the short term; to use parameters you will need to be checking things like heart rate, blood pressure, or blood glucose (sugar) levels more frequently. However, by doing this you may also notice that taking your regular dose as scheduled might not be needed. Your doctor can tell you what the appropriate parameters are for your condition and personal circumstances, and monitoring your numbers closely may mean that you're able to skip and stockpile quite a few doses of your daily medications. Just be sure to refill your prescription at the usual rate, even if you aren't using it all.

4.) Always Say Yes to Antibiotics

Many people have heard that taking antibiotics too frequently can have negative side effects. While this is certainly true, most physicians are still happy to offer and prescribe them if they see a potential need. Things like ear infections, sinus infections, and some minor skin infections are indications for taking antibiotics, however they are also pretty easy to manage without medication and often go away on their own. Never hold off on taking a prescribed antibiotic if your condition is getting worse, but if it seems to be getting better and alternative treatments at home are working, it's likely that you won't need it. If you find yourself in one of these situations and think antibiotics are unnecessary, you're probably right – but you should still see a doctor and if they are willing to write a prescription, take it!

There's no harm in filling an antibiotic prescription as they are generally quite inexpensive with and without insurance, and if you don't end up needing them you will have a nice, unopened course of antibiotics for your stash. It is important to keep in mind that antibiotics are not a one-size-fits-all medication, and certain antibiotics are used for certain problems. A good tip is to write on the bottle what it was prescribed for, and some internet searching can also tell you what other conditions may be treated with that particular antibiotic.

5.) Over the Counter Insulin

This one is for insulin-dependent diabetics specifically, but insulin is of particular importance as managing diabetes is a constant task and even a day or two without needed insulin can be detrimental to one's health. What many people don't know is that some insulin is available without a prescription. These insulins are older, less effective versions of the newer insulins used today, but they are absolutely still effective and better than nothing in a pinch. Pricing for over-the-counter insulin varies, but if you can afford it, it's a great option to have in your stash. Not all pharmacies stock OTC insulin so you'll need to ask around, although Wal-Mart pharmacies are known for having plenty of it. If you do choose to keep a supply of OTC insulin, be sure to consult your doctor as he or she can provide guidance for using those formulas in an emergency.

With these five tips you should be able to get started on building a decent supply of emergency medication. Having a stockpile can provide great peace of mind, and should you ever find yourself unable to refill your medications you can be prepared. Just remember, a medication stash should be tended to regularly, checking for long-past expiration dates and some prescriptions that may have changed according to your condition. Keep instructions for use on all medications, as well as instructions on what to do if you are completely out of medication and have no access to more. Lastly, consider building a great first aid kid as an excellent complement to a medication stockpile! During uncertain times, it is always best to be overprepared.

Medicines that Are Safe to Take After Their Expiration Date

Should we throw away every medication in our homes once they expire? Now that is a question many people have asked and are still asking.

You see, in 1979 the FDA (Food and Drug Administration) passed a law that required every manufacturer to provide a possible expiration date for all medications sold. This date was supposed to guarantee full potency and safety of the drugs. Since then all medications have carried an expiry date. However, the expiration date is only a guarantee from the manufacturer of how long said medication can maintain its stability and potency while in its unopened container. Once the medication is opened, the expiration dates no longer carry much weight.

As a result of the introduction of expiration dates on drugs, billions of dollars have gone down the drain in an effort to get rid of unused expired medications due to possible loss of effectiveness and health risk. This level of wastage inspired a need to investigate the possibility of using said medications even after their expiration date. So the FDA and U.S department of defense carried out a study to test medications' safety and stability after expiration. Prescribed drugs and OTC (over the counter) drugs were tested. This study found that most of the tested medications remained stable and effective beyond their expiration date. In fact, they found out that 90% of the tested expired medications maintained their safety and potency.

According to Francis Flaherty, a former director of the testing programme of FDA, "expiration dates put on by manufacturers, typically have no bearing on whether a drug is usable for longer. A drug maker is required to prove only that a drug is still good on whatever expiration date the company chooses to set. The expiration date doesn't mean, or even suggest, that the drug will stop being effective after that, nor that it will become harmful. Manufacturers put expiration dates on for marketing, rather than scientific reasons. It's not profitable for them to have products on a shelf for 10 years."

Irrespective of this fact, it was also discovered that the forms (liquid or solid) and method of storage (light, heat, humidity, oxygen etc.) influenced the potency of the medications over time. For instance, solid drugs (tablets and capsules) are more stable than liquids (solutions and suspensions) and therefore tend to remain intact and potent long after expiration. Many OTC medications, especially tablets and capsules, remain effective and safe for use after their expiration date.

Ibuprofen tablets, which is a non-steroidal anti-inflammatory drug (NSAIDs), has been found to be potent for 4 to 5 years after opening the container. These medications are used for the relief of moderate pain such as menstrual cramps, joint pains, arthritis, gout attacks etc. In cases of a fever they can function as antipyretic drugs.

Tylenol or acetaminophen doubles both as an antipyretic medication to treat fevers and as an analgesic to treat mild to moderate pains such as headaches. Studies have shown that Tylenol or acetaminophen can maintain its potency for up to 4 or 5 years of having opened the container. Liquid forms of acetaminophen should be used by the expiration date since liquid forms deteriorate faster than solid ones.

Aspirin or acetylsalicylic acid has proven to remain potent within 5 years of opening. Aspirin also belongs to the NSAIDs family but aside functioning as an anti-inflammatory drug, it functions as an analgesic, antipyretic and antiplatelet medication. However, one side effect of aspirin is bleeding, therefore utmost care must be taken with the consumption of this medication.

Anti-histamine tablets such as loratadine (second generation antihistamine) and diphenhydramine (first generation antihistamine) are very efficient for treating and managing allergies, such as hay fever and skin allergies. Based on studies carried out, antihistaminic drugs can be used for over 5 years after opening.

Other medications are advised to be used before or by their expiration dates.

Antibiotics, which are excellent medications for treating bacterial infections, are prescribed for a full course which means there should be no left overs. Both liquid and solid forms of antibiotics should be consumed by the expiration date.

Cough syrups have components that break up easily and do not remain stable over a long period of time, therefore it's recommended that you consume cough syrups before their expiration date.

Nasal syrups have certain preservatives that make them safe to use, however these preservatives degrade overtime reducing the safety of the syrup after a long period of time. Use your nasal syrup before expiration.

Eye drops are liquid medicines and so can easily get contaminated and because the eye is a very sensitive organ, it is advisable to dispose of expired eye drops. Use them as prescribed and before expiration.

Insulin, vaccines, and epi pens must be replaced once expired as they tend to degrade quickly over a period of time.

OTC or prescribed sleeping pills and valium lose their potency overtime making patients to take more pills to achieve same effect and thereby leading to overdose or addiction. These sleeping pills and valium must be used within one year of opening.

Prescription drugs like Adderall and Mydayis should be taken according to physician's instructions and also within one year of opening. The loss of potency over time can interfere with its function in cases of ADHD.

In as much as most medications remain potent and effective past their expiration date, it's important to store medications in the right environments to maintain their potency. Do not store medications in the bathroom as the heat and humidity from the hot water shower can destroy drug's potency. Always store drugs in cool and dry places away from children's reach.

Remember to close medicine containers properly after use. Frequently check your medications for signsof deterioration such as discoloration, powdery texture, bad smell and in cases of liquid medications, look out for cloudy or filmy solutions and suspensions.

Remember, if you have any doubts regarding the consumption of expired medications, consult a physician or a pharmacist.

The Biggest Mistakes You Can Make in a Blackout

Electricity is a basic life necessity. Many of life's processes are powered by electricity. Food and water require electricity to remain intact. Electricity has been used over the years to pump water, store food and medications, generate heat, generate cold, make certain devices work and illuminate spaces. However, heavy rains, thunderstorms, hurricanes etc. tend to interrupt electricity functions especially when they result in a blackout. Blackouts can last for few minutes, sometimes hours, and other times for days. A power outage is an unpredictable event, which means we must be prepared for such. Knowing what not to do and what to do in a blackout is essential to survive one.

Most people make mistakes that could cost them their life in a blackout. Some of the frequent mistakes people make in a blackout putting their health, and therefore their life, at risk are:

1. Emergency Kit

Most people do not have an emergency kit in their homes in case of a disaster. In a blackout, accidents are bound to happen; there could be cuts or scrapes. An emergency kit will come in handy.

Your emergency kit should contain certain over the counter medications that can be useful in a disaster, such as acetaminophen, Ibuprofen, and oral rehydration solution. Other medications such as medications for chronic diseases like diabetes, high blood pressure, Asthma etc. must be readily available in your emergency kit if you have family members suffering from these illnesses. Other things you should have in your kit are a first aid kit, flash lights, extra batteries, perishable foods, extra water, and blankets.

2. A Backup Oxygen Tank

Administering oxygen to sick people at home has been made easy with the help of oxygen concentrators. Oxygen concentrators are used in patients who suffer from breathing difficulty, such as in Asthma, COPD (chronic obstructive pulmonary disease), lung cancer, COVID 19 etc. Oxygen concentrators function by pulling the air around us and filtering the nitrogen content before administering it to the patient. The downside however is that they run on electricity, which means in the case of a power outage, the patient will not receive oxygen and this could lead to complications and death. Having a backup oxygen tank is necessary to avoid depriving patients of oxygen as a result of a blackout. Oxygen tanks administer liquid oxygen to the patient manually without the use of electricity and so they are the best thing that can happen to an oxygen-dependent patient in a blackout.

3. A Backup Generator

In the US and many other countries, most patients and the elderly are no longer being hospitalized for long periods or sent to nursing homes for care, as studies have shown that they thrive better around family members.

Most of these patients require long term treatments through medical devices that obviously need to be plugged in to electricity. Since these devices are now portable and can be installed in the homes of patients, they receive their treatments at home. Some of these devices are CPAP (continuous positive airway pressure), BiPAP (bi-level positive airway pressure), dialysis devices, power wheel chair, electric beds, oxygen concentrators etc.

In a blackout, these devices shut down and can no longer function which is a very good reason to have a backup generator at home. With a backup generator, even in the event of a power outage, these medical devices can still work.

4. Charcoal Grills and Stoves

In winter, a power outage can lead to very low temperature which is very uncomfortable. In order to heat their homes, some people use charcoal grills or stoves. This is a very dangerous practice as these equipments release carbon monoxides into your living space.

Carbon monoxide poisoning (CMP) can lead to tissue damage and death. When a large amount of carbon monoxide is inhaled, it enters into the bloodstream and displaces oxygen, meaning our body gets blood and carbon monoxide but not oxygen, which of course is deadly. And because carbon monoxide is an odorless gas, it is difficult to detect its presence in your home. CMP can cause tension headaches, dizziness, nausea, vomiting, confusion etc. Beware of these symptoms.

5. Downed Wires

If you are outside your home during a power outage, avoid touching any and all downed wires as these can still have live energy in them leading to electrical injuries. Electrical injuries will vary based on the path of the electric current. Having contact with a live downed wire can cause burns, respiratory arrest, cardiac damage, brain injuries, and death. Make sure to avoid any downed wire in a blackout.

6. Candles

Lighting a candle is the first response to the absence of electricity irrespective of the cause of the blackout. Whether the blackout will only last for few minutes or for hours or days, it is not recommended to light candles in these situations. Candles are highly flammable and can easily be knocked down thereby starting a fire. A fire can cause smoke inhalation, second- or third-degree burns, death and destruction of properties. If you must use candles, place them in a protective container and keep an eye on them or better still, use battery powered LED lights and flash lights.

7. Medication that Requires Refrigeration

Throwing away medications that require refrigeration is a waste and puts the health of the patient at risk. An important thing to note is that these medications can be safely stored in the event of a blackout, without losing their effectiveness or potency.

To keep medications such as insulin, humira, eye drops, and vaccines safe and effective, maintain the fridge closed; a closed fridge will keep these medications intact for 2 – 3 hours. If a longer blackout is expected, take out these medications immediately and place them in an ice chest or a cooler packed with ice or cold packs. Make sure the medications are not directly in contact with the ice, wrap them with paper or towel to avoid freezing. Frozen medications lose their potency and effectiveness. Remember to use a thermometer to check the temperature within the ice chest.

In addition, most Insulins now come in vials that remain intact opened or unopened outside the fridge. They can stay outside the fridge for 4 weeks and not lose their potency.

We never know how long a blackout is going to last, so not being prepared is the greatest mistake you can make. Not being prepared can cost you your health and that of your loved ones. Not being prepared can lead to complications of chronic conditions and death. Staying prepared is the best thing you can do for you and your loved ones. Stay prepared.

The Only 4 Antibiotics People Should Stockpile

Antibiotics will become priceless in times of need once they become scarce. Having these four at home for you and your family is at least as important as having food stockpiles. But under no circumstance should you take them without consulting a doctor first.

Knowing about certain animal antibiotics can come in handy when and only if the need arises. For instance, in the case of a shortage of medications or in cases where people run out of their medication and require urgent treatment, these medications might be very helpful.

During the pandemic people died not just from the virus but from lack of access to healthcare centers and medications. People ran out of medications, others got sick but could not access hospitals or pharmacies; in such cases certain over the counter veterinary drugs can save a life.
It's been said that humans are simply higher animals and regardless of our differences, we share a lot of similarities with animals. One of the so many things we have in common is health.

Animals suffer from certain diseases that humans suffer from as well, such as mastitis, digestive infections, respiratory infections, abscesses, etc. Likewise, they also require treatment just like humans do. One of the frequently used medications in animals are antibiotics which are used mainly for three reasons: therapeutic reasons, prevention of diseases (prophylaxis), and to promote growth in animals. Animals also require regular health checkups by a veterinarian, just as humans require the same from a physician. Based on the veterinarian's examination a medication can be prescribed if need be.

However, there are certain veterinary medications that are over the counter and do not require prescription. Antibiotics treat bacterial infections whether it is an infection in the human body or an animal body. So, the same antibiotics will function both in animals and humans alike.

The function of an antibiotic is to destroy bacteria either by stunting their growth or by directly killing them. This function remains the same, whether they are acting on a human body or an animal body. Yet due to differences in the gut system of animals and humans, animals might tolerate certain antibiotics better than humans and for that reason, certain medications specify animal use only.

There are some over the counter veterinary antibiotics that can be used in humans in extreme cases, when the need arises. Nonetheless, it is important that you consult your physician before taking any of these four veterinary antibiotics.

Azithromycin is an antimicrobial drug that belongs to the family of the macrolides, containing an active ingredient called azithromycin. It is used in the treatment of respiratory infections such as pneumonia, pharyngitis, and tonsillitis in humans. It can also be used to treat uncomplicated skin infections caused by staphylococcus aureus, genital ulcers, urethritis, and cervicitis in women. In the case of a shortage or in an emergency where there is no access to azithromycin, a veterinary over the counter antibiotic called Eritromycin, which belongs to the same family of drugs, can be taken as a replacement.

Doxycycline is an antibiotic of the tetracycline family; it is used in humans to treat a variety of bacterial infections such as pneumonias, skin infections, urinary tract infections, STIs (sexually transmitted infections) and in the prevention of malaria. However, in the absence of this drug, Tetracycline, which is used in treating infections in poultry, cattle, sheep, and swine can come in handy to replace doxycycline.

Neomycin is used in the treatment of bacterial gastrointestinal infections in cattle, sheep and goats. It belongs to a family of antibiotics called aminoglycosides and can be used in the place of other aminoglycoside family members such as gentamycin and amikacin. Gentamicin and amikacin are effective in treating abdominal and urinary tract infections and are also used in the treatment and prophylaxis of endocarditis in humans. However, precaution must be taken as aminoglycosides in excess dosage can lead to renal failure or deafness.

Lincomycin belongs to the lincosamide group antibiotics. It is used in animals such as dogs, cats, pigs, and birds to treat gram positive infections. It can be used in the absence of clindamycin, which is used in treating the following conditions in humans: skin and soft tissue infections, osteomyelitis, septic arthritis, acute sinusitis, pharyngitis, and otitis media.

It is important to note that the above-mentioned medications will only treat infections caused by bacteria. They are useless in the presence of infections caused by viruses such as a cold or flu. Also taking into consideration that every antibiotic has adverse effects, it is imperative that you consult your physician for an accurate diagnosis before consuming any of the above-mentioned drugs. If you run out of medications and have any of these veterinary drugs in your home, please consult your physician before consumption.

MENTAL HEALTH

Mental health is a state of psychological and emotional well-being that is easily influenced by the environment. Our emotional strength or lability depends on many factors. In recent years, elements such as the social environment at home and at work and even the climate have been studied as important to our state of mind and perception of things.

We have changes in our behavior on a daily basis depending on the situations we face during the day. Thus, we can feel happy, angry, and sad on the same day without that meaning that there is any problem with our mental health.

Situations that put us in a high level of stress activate the fight or flight response, which includes important drastic changes in our mental health state. Circumstances that present themselves unexpectedly that we don't know how to cope with can usually trigger stress responses.

New situations, diseases, bad news, and worrisome world information, such as fires, environmental pollution, deaths, or famine, are facts that alter our mental state to a greater or lesser degree. Some people tolerate the changes that come through worrying better than others. Just as there are people who have higher thresholds for pain, there are those who can tolerate a higher level of stress.

Stress can present itself in different ways depending on biological and environmental factors.

It is sometimes difficult for people to notice a change in their usual behavior. Changes as subtle as feeling bored or not wanting to do anything, being sleepier than usual, or not finding fun in activities that normally entertain us are warning signs that something is disturbing our mental health.

No one is prepared to face every scenario simply because some are unfamiliar. If we have never had to be in that situation, we won't know how to deal with it. Facing these new events will generate changes to which we can adapt as much as possible.

The most common mental health issues are: stress, depression, anxiety, and dementia.

1. STRESS

Stress is the physical response to a tense situation. This response occurs due to the hormones that are released in the face of the situation we detect as "dangerous." It is a normal physiological reaction that may be beneficial and necessary at some times but causes discomfort and unpleasantness at others.

Feelings of sadness, anger, and worry, among others, are manifestations of this tension. Other types of symptoms, such as insomnia, muscle contractions, headaches, abdominal cramping, and diarrhea, are also a presentation of stress.

Stress is present in our lives from birth. When the fetus passes through the birth canal, a strong response is generated that helps to activate the descending movements and start the breathing process. Later in life, we respond better or worse to different situations depending on the impact they have on us. Perhaps before an important interview or exam, you have had a stomachache or back pain. These symptoms are caused by the body in response to the stress.

There are people who cannot adequately handle stressful situations, and in some cases, they must be hospitalized or taken to mental clinics for rest.

What Symptoms Can Intense Stress Cause?

Momentary loss of vision, speech, or hearing is one of the most alarming symptoms of an extreme state of stress. In these cases, you should try to stay calm, and the symptom will disappear completely after a few minutes.

If you are a nervous person by nature, it is important that you practice relaxation techniques. At the end of this chapter, you will find some guided relaxation exercises that can help you cope with daily stress and improve in extraordinary situations.

2. DEPRESSION

Depression is a state of mind characterized by deep, often unexplained sadness that impairs our ability to perform daily activities. The male to female ratio presentation is 1:2. It should not be confused with "being sad," since depression goes beyond that and does not improve as a result of a behavioral change on the part of the person concerned.

It is important to recognize the changes in behavior that occur gradually in a person who is depressed since in its early stages, it can be treated with therapies that can be carried out at home.

Symptoms and Signs

- **Mood:** anxiety, general discontent, guilt, hopelessness, loss of interest or pleasure in activities, mood swings like sadness or anger, among others
- **Behavioral:** agitation, unusual crying, irritability, social isolation
- **Changes in sleep patterns:** early awakening, excess sleepiness or insomnia, restless sleep
- **Changes in dietary patterns:** excessive hunger or loss of appetite
- **Cognitive:** lack of concentration, slowness in activity

The best way to recognize depress is with the mnemonic **SIG E CAPS**:

Sleep (Am I sleeping too much or less than normal?)

Interest (loss of interest or pleasure in activities)

Guilt (feelings of worthlessness or inappropriate guilt)

Energy (decreased or fatigued)

Concentration (decreased concentration) **A**ppetite

(increased or decreased appetite/weight)

Psychomotor (agitation or slower movements)

Suicidal ideation

Diagnosis requires a depressed mood or anhedonia (loss of interest/pleasure) abd > or = 5 of the signs and symptoms from the "SIG E CAPS" mnemonic. If you recognize some of these signs in yourself or in a family member or neighbor, you or they are likely to be in a state of depression.

Relaxation techniques and breathing exercises are treatments that can be used as an alternative therapy to drugs for this type of disorder.

SKIN AND SKIN APPENDAGES

Before the third year of medical training, I didn't know that the skin was an organ; in fact, it's the largest organ of the body and constitutes the first barrier of defense against microorganisms and traumas. It is considered a neurological organ since it has nerve endings that allow us to communicate with the environment.

It also has the function of lowering body temperature through sweating. In addition, through its changes, we can guide the diagnosis of many skin and non-skin conditions. Its changes in color, odor, and texture are good indicators of a number of systemic diseases.

The cutaneous annexes are complementary structures to the skin that protrude from it. They include body hair, nails, and sweat glands.

The easiest way to keep skin in good condition is to keep it clean and moisturized. Cleaning should be done with a special soap for this purpose. In my case, I always use specific face care products. These types of soaps are milder and adjust to the pH and moisture of the skin.

In my country, it is very common to use a laundry soap bar to clean infected skin, as if it had bacteriostatic properties.

It is so common, that when a patient with a wound or allergy arrives to the hospital, it should be specified that they should not wash with "Jabón Las Llaves," which is a local brand so well known that any soap bars are called by that name.

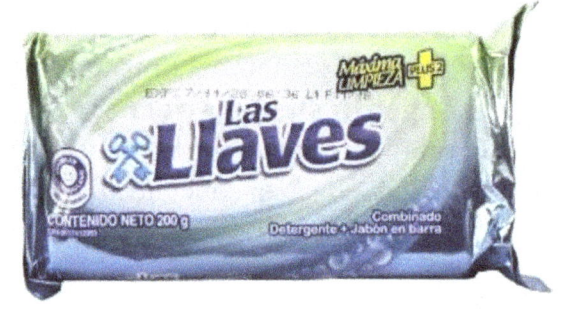

This soap has been traditional throughout Venezuelasince 1877. I cannot say when it became part of wound care in popular culture, but I do know that it is deeply rooted, especially in the interior of the country.

If you've ever wondered what it would be like to bathe with a laundry soap bar, you have to know they have very alkaline detergents that alter the surface layer of the skin, making it susceptible to damage.

Instead of providing the correct moist and oily environment, it dries out the skin.

If you are allergic or you get skin reactions easily, it is best to use hypoallergenic or non-detergent soaps.

Moisturizing the skin is easy. Just by staying well hydrated, we already have 80% of the work done. You'll complete the other 20% by applying a moisturizing cream, preferably unscented or soft or some natural oil.

Dermatologists, as well as many models and artists, always share a useful tip that helps them to better absorb the moisturizer. This is to apply it after a shower or bath, when the skin is still wet.

Some people, though, do not like the wet feeling that the application of the moisturizer leaves. However, there are many products available that dry almost immediately without leaving any residue.

I always use moisturizing body cream, day and night facial cream, and eye and under-eye cream. I am a bit obsessive about using them because taking care of our skin is what gives it elasticity and a healthy look.

I have a ritual in which I use a specific product with charcoal to clean my face, and after drying well without rubbing the towel, I apply the corresponding face cream. I only use the eye cream at night.

After bathing, I use moisturizer, and once a week, I like to use essential oil of coconut or almonds, which helps maintain the normal oily layer of the skin. When I can't put cream on, I feel my skin is very dry. That's why I recommend its daily use as that sticky feeling is only at the beginning.

It is important to say that the care of the skin is for both men and women.

WHAT DERMATOLOGICAL PRODUCTS SHOULD I HAVE AT HOME?

Neutral soap for cleaning hands and body is a must. Remember that if for any reason you must wash your hands frequently, there may be a tendency toward dryness of the skin, so it is important to have a moisturizing cream on hand.

Sunscreen is important, with SPF over 30 in the summer. Also, special skin moisturizers for the winter can prevent cracking and small wounds that can cause inflammation and infection.

An antibiotic cream is also useful. There are many brands sold over the counter, but the active ingredients are almost always the same: *Bacitracin* or *Mupirocin*.

Products that contain many compounds combined, such as steroids and antifungals, are not recommended as they tend to mask some conditions and make them worse over time.

It is best to buy a specific product for each disease. In the end, it is more cost effective than having to go to the dermatologist for an advanced disease.

The most common skin diseases are: corns, warts, burns and scalds, dermatitis, fungal infections, insect bites and stings, cellulitis and abscesses, ulcers, open wounds, and nail trauma.

1. CORNS

Corns are calluses that form on the toes over the joints. They can become very uncomfortable when fully developed and can become inflamed, ulcerated, bloody, and infected.

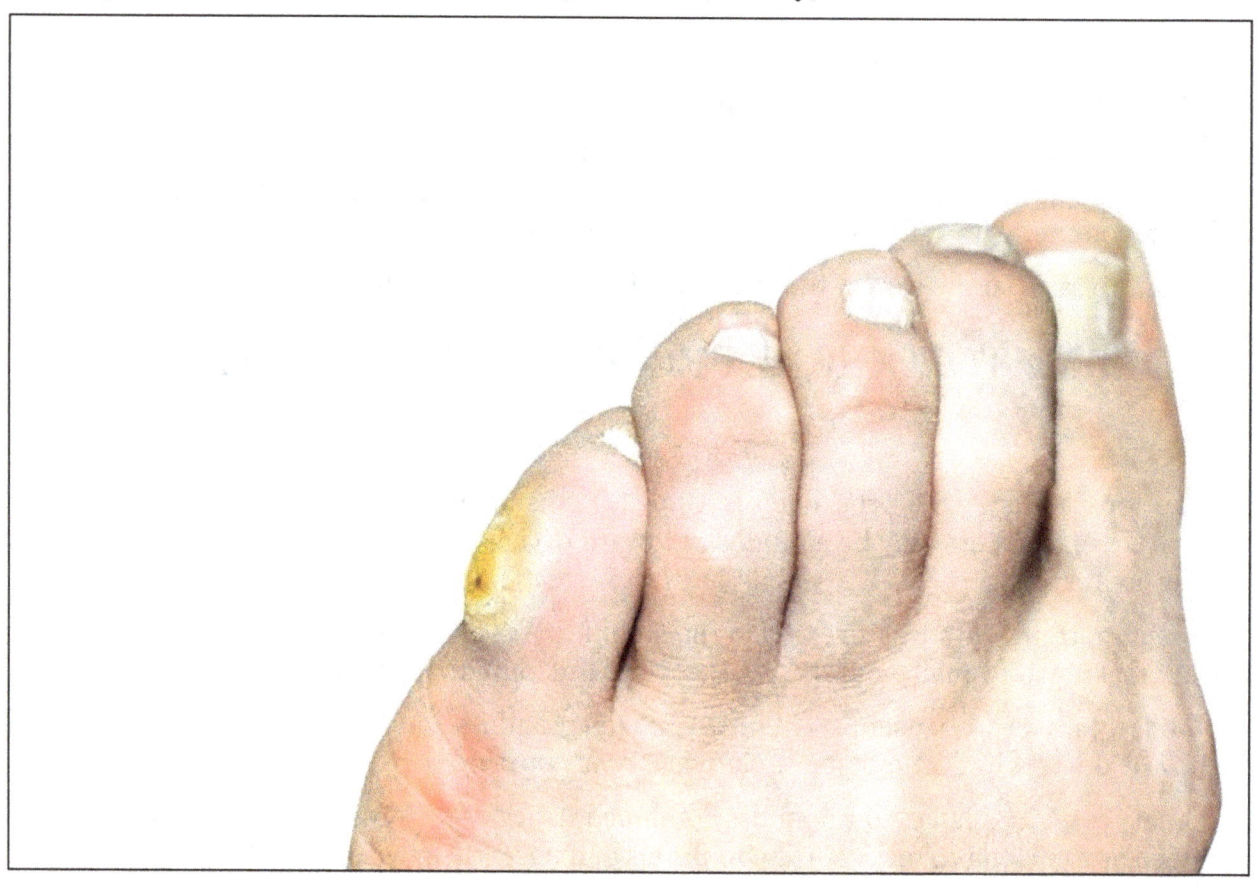

The best way to prevent their development is to use moisturizing cream and a pumice stone and to wear comfortable footwear.

When these measures are not enough, it is convenient to have some corn plasters at home, but if you do not have this, there is nothing to worry about. The corn plaster is nothing more than a small cylinder that forms a cushion between the shoe and the corn, smeared with a little solution of acetyl salicylic acid that is supposed to reduce inflammation and diminish the corn. The main objective of the treatment is to avoid ulcers since wounded skin can easily lead to infections.

When it is not possible to go to a pharmacy to buy these types of items, measures such as dipping your feet in warm water for ten minutes daily or every two days can be used to improve the condition of the thickened skin.

Moisturizing cream or Vaseline are great tools to help as well as wearing comfortable footwear, if possible of a type that is not closed or has enough space at the top.

Infection is easily recognized when the skin of the affected toe is red and warmer compared to the temperature of the rest of the foot, either with or without discharge.

2. WARTS

A wart is an abnormal growth on the skin, commonly found on the palms and soles, that is characterized by a painless, cauliflower-shaped lesion.

It usually has no major complications, although rubbing can make it lose the top layer of skin that covers it, leading to uncomfortable symptoms. It can also become ulcerated and trigger skin infections.

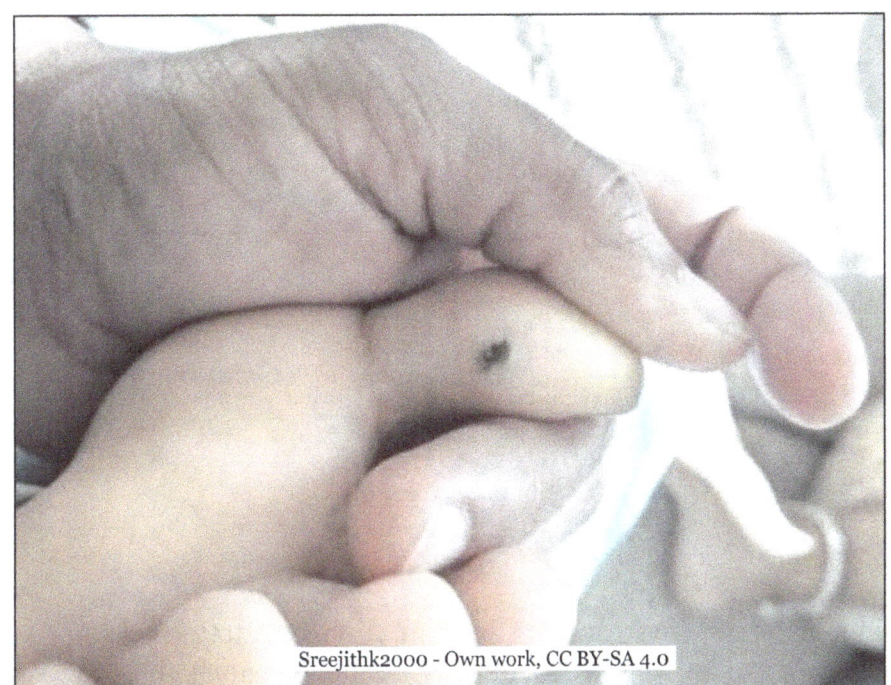
Sreejithk2000 - Own work, CC BY-SA 4.0

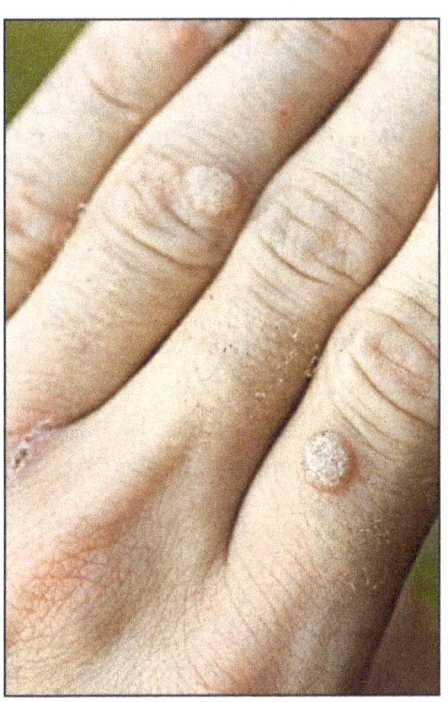

3. INSECT BITES AND STINGS

We are exposed to insect bites and stings at all times. These injuries are usually mild and sometimes go unnoticed. Insect bites are usually very itchy because they create an allergic reaction on the skin. There are people who are much more sensitive to some bites and stings; in these cases, you have to be very careful and watch out for any symptoms.

Treatment of a sting is simple and relies on the application of topical creams or lotions to improve symptoms. Calamine lotion usually provides significant relief from itching and gives a cool sensation to the skin. However, it is best to use a cream with corticosteroids that help reduce inflammation and improve redness.

Itching can become a very annoying symptom, so it is recommended to take antihistamines for three days (Zyrtec or Chlor-Trimeton). The vast majority of insect bite cases are resolved within a few days without major complications.

When Should I Worry?

When the bite is on the face, we must be aware of the changes that occur in the patient, especially if it is near the eyes or in the so-called "danger triangle".

Patients who are allergic to food, dust, and other agents are often also susceptible to stings.

In these cases, it is important to notice if the person manifests any respiratory symptoms in the first hour after the sting.

<u>*If the sting was made by a scorpion:*</u> Most scorpions do not produce much damage, but some contain venom that is very toxic to humans. Therefore, it is important to closely monitor a person who has been stung by a scorpion.

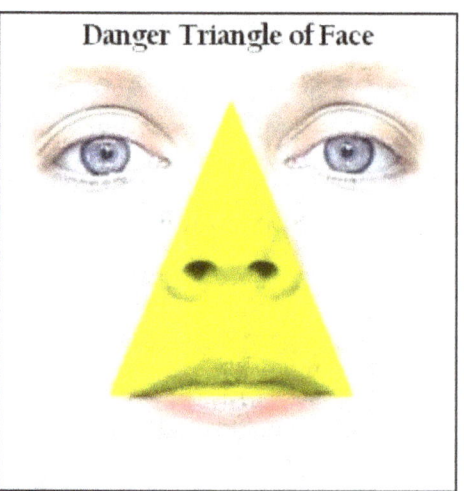
Danger Triangle of Face

Warning Signs

- Difficulty in breathing
- Sudden increase in heart rate
- Swollen lips and face
- Numbness of the skin
- Nausea.

How Can I Be Prepared?

It is absolutely necessary to have an epinephrine self-injector pen (Epi-Pen, Auvi-Q, Adrenaclick). This instrument can save lives in the event of an anaphylactic reaction. Whether you can get help or not, the seconds saved by an epinephrine injection are very valuable and can define the boundary between life and death.

The epinephrine auto-injector consists of a pencil that comes loaded with enough adrenaline for one patient. All you have to do is remove the safety catch and press the pencil on the middle of the thigh, and the injection will be triggered.

Once injected, the patient should improve within the next half hour. If the symptoms continue, a second injection can be given.

Ninety-five percent of cases that do not respond completely to the first dose will respond to the second. If you are able to seek specialized help by this time, explain the number of injections given and the symptoms the patient had. If not, continue strict monitoring of that person for at least 24 hours.

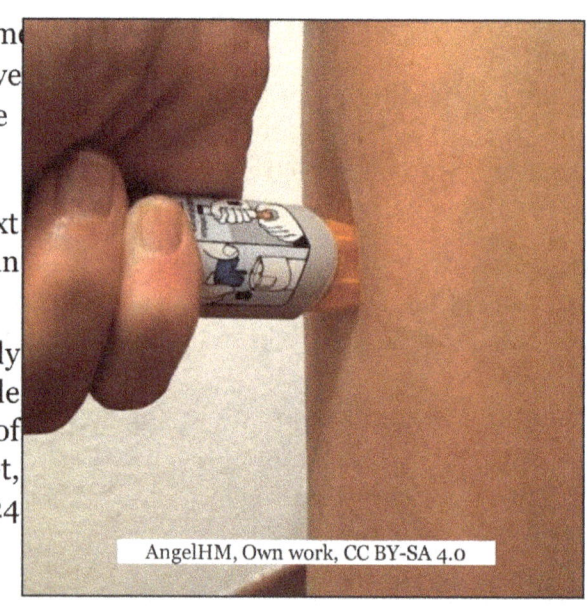
AngelHM, Own work, CC BY-SA 4.0

4. NAIL TRAUMA

Trauma to the nail can occur by various mechanisms. The main one is a **blow** that, when strong enough, causes bleeding in the nail bed and the nail looks a little purple. When there is **repeated trauma**, as in the case of dancers, professional football players, and runners, the nails can be deformed.

Another mechanism of trauma, very common in children, is nail biting. This habit results in softening of the nail, loss of cuticle, and contamination that can be very serious and difficult to manage.

What Can I Do at Home?

It is rare that trauma to the nail is severe enough to require emergency assistance. Most nail problems can be handled easily at home. If there is a bruise under the nail on the nail bed and it causes pain or a lot of pressure, you can drain it. You don't have to use a scalpel to do this. With the help of a sterile needle, you can use the one in a syringe, you'll be fine.

The most important thing is to leave your finger soaking for 10 minutes in warm water. This step is essential to make the nail softer and the bruise more liquid. If the nail has come off completely or almost completely, try sticking it back on top of the bed with adhesive around it. This technique has two objectives: one is to serve as a guide for the new nail that will come out, and the other is not to lose the space of the nail, which, when empty, can form skin and scar.

Ingrown Toenails (Onychocryptosis)

Onychrocryptosis is a very common pathology. Although I have never suffered from it, I have had several cases, including a colleague at the hospital and several military personnel in Amazonas. In this condition, the nail grows abnormally, cutting one side of the nail bed and getting into the skin.

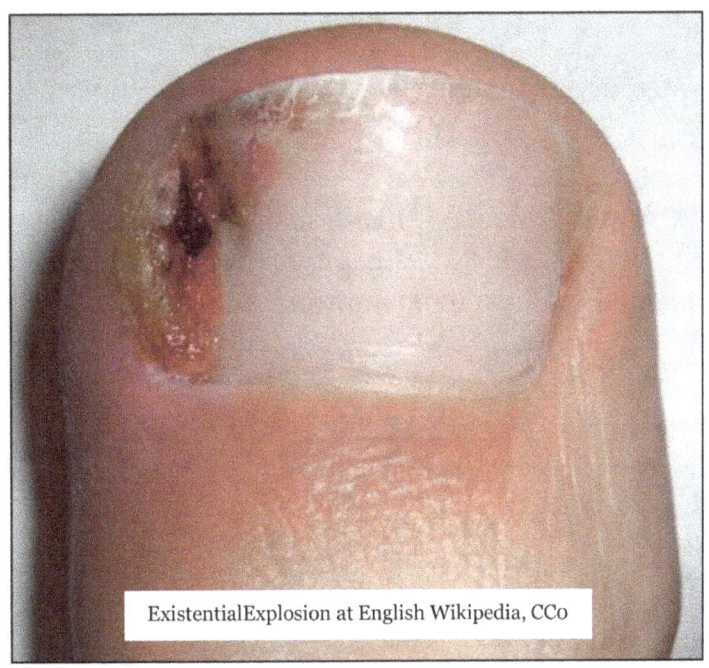

ExistentialExplosion at English Wikipedia, CC0

This situation, besides being painful, usually causes the contamination of the affected finger, so the patient seeks to cut out only the part of the nail that is embedded in the skin for a temporary improvement.

Dealing Effectively with Ingrown Nails Without Leaving Home

In order to break the cycle of the ingrown nail, it is necessary to perform a procedure that, although a little painful, is very effective.

The first thing I like to do when I have to perform a surgical procedure on inflamed skin is to indicate antibiotic and anti-inflammatory for a few days, which assures me that the healing will be better and the surgical procedure will be well tolerated by the patient.

In the case of onychocryptosis, if the toe is inflamed and sensitive with discharge coming out of the sides, I indicate Ciprofloxacin 500mg every 12 hours for 10 days and Ibuprofen 200mg every 8 hours for 5 days. On the fifth day of the antibiotic, I check the condition of the foot, and usually it is time to perform this technique.

The idea of the procedure is to remove the ingrown piece of nail from the skin and cut it down to the base so that it does not grow back in that direction. It is a very effective technique that prevents the nail from growing back ingrown in many cases.

If it happens again, the nail must be completely removed so that a new one grows in. This should be supervised by the specialist who will work so that it does not deviate from its direction.

Step 1

The first thing you do is soak the affected foot in a solution of warm water and soap for 15 minutes.

Step 2

Remove the foot from the water, dry it well and clean the toe with alcohol.

Step 3

With a rubber band, make a firm tourniquet at the base of the affected toe to decrease sensation and prevent bleeding. At this point, you can apply anesthetic cream or spray. Remember that this procedureis painful, but the benefit is incredible and the relief immediate.

Step 4

Look for the upper edge of the ingrown nail and pull it out of the skin over its full vertical length. This can be done with a sharp instrument such as a thick needle. Even flossing works to effectively pull out that piece of nail.

Step 5

With scissors or a scalpel blade, cut that piece of nail lengthwise, including the base.

Clean the bed well, which may have traces of pus in it. Remove the band from the base of the toe or finger.

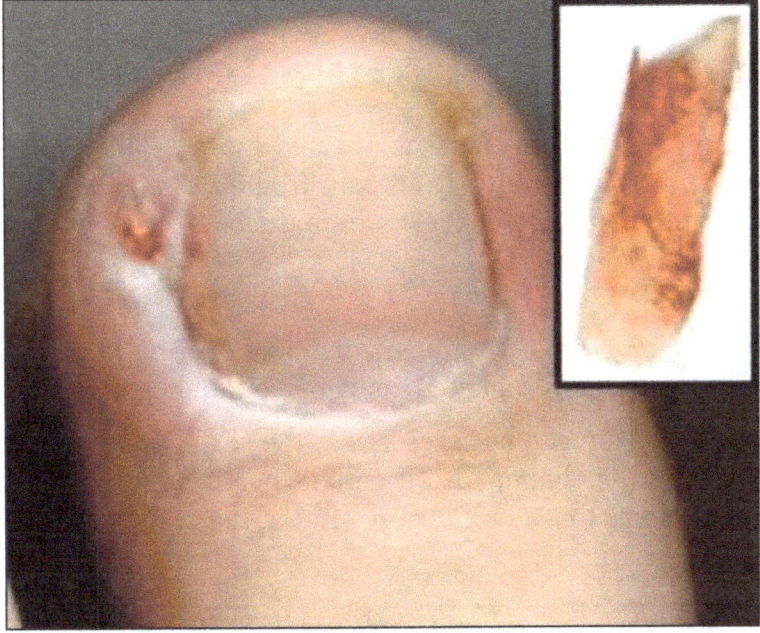

The procedure is completed by suturing the skin to make the surface flatter. However, this can wait for a consultation with a specialist.

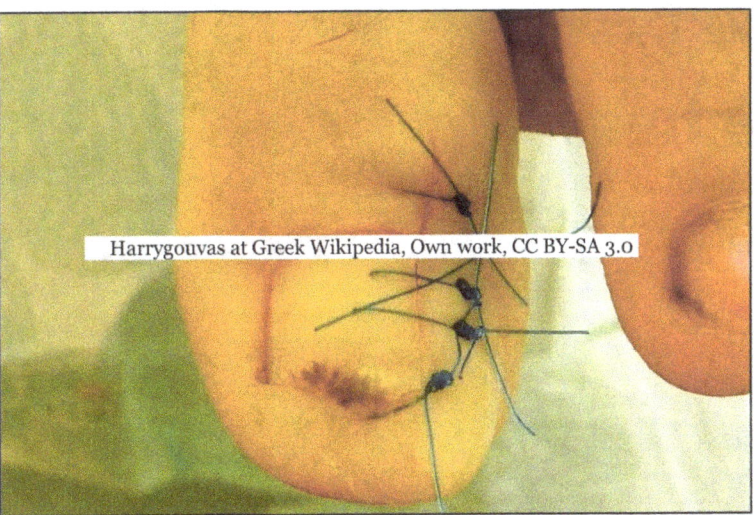

With the technique described, the pain improves 100% as well as the infection, partially curing the patient who, hopefully, will not have recurrences in the future. If it happens again, this procedure can be done again, and it is necessary to go to the specialist when possible to have it completed.

 Antibiotic treatment should be continued for the remaining five days and the region operated on should be cleaned daily with alcohol. Also, for one week, wear comfortable or open shoes.

HEAD AND NECK

1. Headaches and Muscle Contractures

Headaches are a very common symptom that has affected most people, both children and adults, at some point. Its causes are diverse and range from pain from stress or tension to vascular conditions. Headaches can also be a symptom of a problem elsewhere, such as the sinuses, neck, or spine.

Types of Headaches

Headaches are classified as *primary* or *secondary* depending on whether they originate as an isolated disease or are an expression of another problem. Ninety percent of headaches are primary and benign.

In other words, even though the pain can be severe, as in the case of migraine, it is not caused by a life-threatening condition. On the other hand, the secondary headache manifests itself as a symptom of another disease. Most are problems that can improve without major complications, such as neck muscle contracture or sinus congestion.

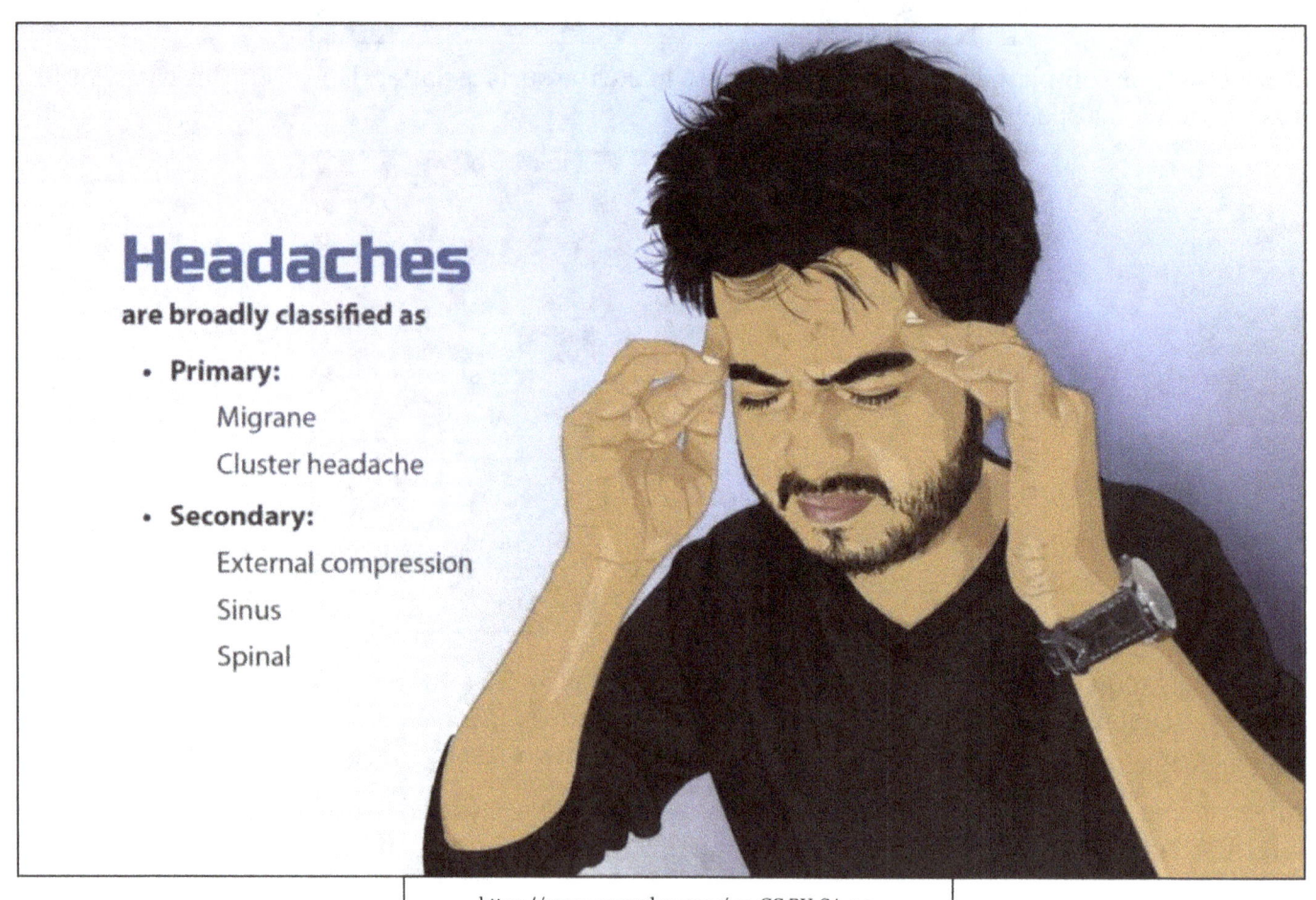

https://www.myupchar.com/en, CC BY-SA 4.0

a) Primary Headaches

Migraine is the most common type of headache. Most of us have had a migraine attack at some point. This type of pain is characterized by being strong and having a series of symptoms that accompany it, making it a real, often disabling condition.

Migraine is subdivided into more than two hundred types, according to the characteristics of the pain. The most common are *migraine with aura* (complicated migraine), *migraine without aura* (common migraine), and *chronic migraine*.

When we talk about aura, we are referring to a series of sensory events that can precede the intense headache of migraine. Some people report a sound seeing a bright halo around things, or even a different smell before the headache.

Thus, a person who suffers migraine attacks with aura is able to recognize the arrival of one of these events by feeling the previous symptoms.

Migraine without aura is the most common. It is a severe headache that can last from a few hours to a couple of days. It is accompanied by photophobia, nausea, and vomiting.

Cluster headache is one of the most painful headaches that a person can experience. It presents as a brief, excruciating, unilateral headache around the eyes. They normally last around thirty minutes to three hours.

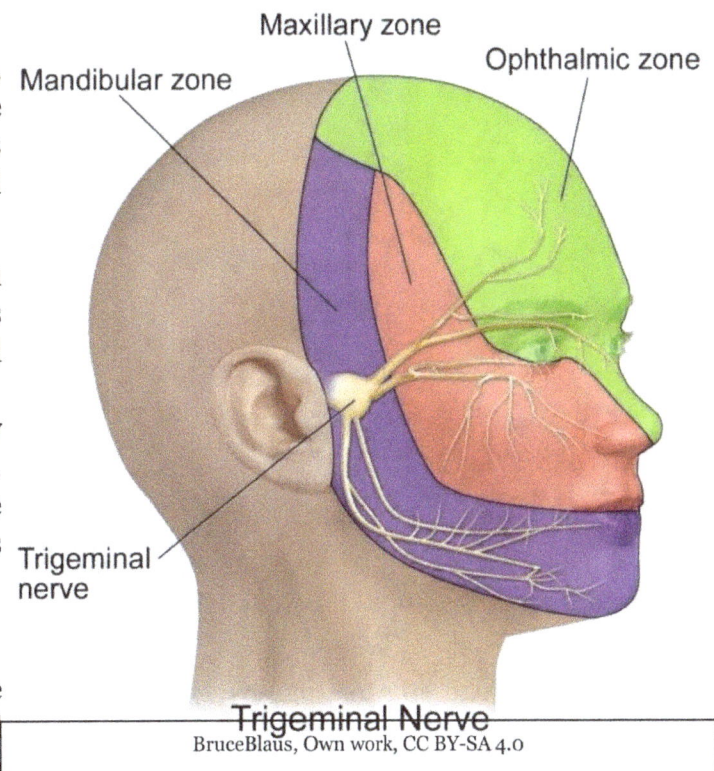

Trigeminal Nerve
BruceBlaus, Own work, CC BY-SA 4.0

They generally come as clusters of time, affecting the same part of the head at the same time of the day (commonly during sleep). It is associated with runny nose, lacrimation, and red eyes.

Tension-type headache is the most common type of headache diagnosed in adults. It presents with a tight, band-like pain around the head triggered frequently by fatigue or stress.
Anxiety, poor concentration, and difficulty sleeping may also be seen accompanying it. Relaxation, massages, hot baths, and avoidance of stressors are the first recommendations given to these patients.

Trigeminal neuralgia

The trigeminal is a cranial nerve that has three branches that are distributed between the skull and the face. Its inflammation produces an intense, very annoying pain.

Many refer to it as one of the strongest burning pains they have ever felt. It is not the most frequent condition, but it does occur, mainly in the elderly.

b) Secondary Headaches

Cervicogenic Headache

This term refers to headaches caused by tension of the muscles of the neck and spine as well as those of the occipital region of the skull. The headache is intense and similar to a migraine; in fact, it is very difficult to differentiate them. Some of the factors that contribute to the appearance of this type of headache are stress, eyestrain, tiredness, and trauma.

It is important to differentiate it from migraine because the treatment is different. Although both improve with the administration of analgesics, in the case of contracture of the muscles, a muscle relaxant and other therapies, such as massage and meditation, should be added.

Sinus Headache

Sinus congestion, or sinusitis, is one of the conditions most often associated with headaches. It is easyto differentiate from a migraine because it occurs in patients who are allergic or who have a process that involves a lot of mucous secretion through the nose and mouth. The sensation is one of strong pressure on the face and the front of the head and may be associated with fever, sore throat, and earache.

1. **Frontal sinuses**
2. **Ethmoid sinuses**
3. **Sphenoid sinuses**
4. **Maxillary sinuses**

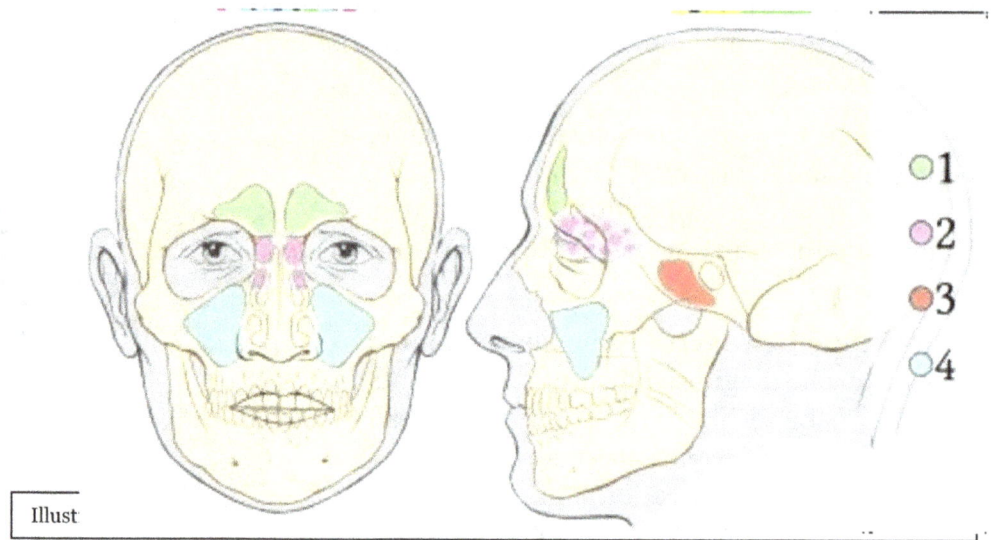

Illust

Hypertension Headache

Increased blood pressure is a cause of headaches that can lead to serious complications. Many patients are hypertensive and do not know it, so they do not receive treatment.

Although headaches are not a specific symptom of hypertension, when a headache occurs in a patient suffering from high blood pressure, it should be treated immediately as it is a complication.

Hypertension is often called a "silent killer" because it can remain silent for years as the body adapts to these high blood pressure values. This is why we can find patients with exaggeratedly high blood pressure levels who did not know they were suffering from hypertension.

I recommend having a blood pressure monitor as there is no other way to know this number.

Treatment Options

Headaches usually get better with common painkillers. NSAIDs work very well in those who are not allergic and do not have a chronic condition.

The combination of acetaminophen, aspirin, and caffeine (Excedrin Migraine) has a very good tolerance and lessens pain because this medicine adds the effect of caffeine, which contracts the blood vessels, to the analgesic effect of the aspirin and acetaminophen.

Lifestyle changes should be taken into account to prevent headaches. Avoiding situations of stress and tension sometimes is necessary as these can be triggers for the pain.

On the migraine subject, I have a lot of experience since I have been suffering from migraines for many years. Although they have improved over time, I occasionally encounter this unpleasant pain again.

My triggers were sleeplessness, long hours without food, and red wine. It was important for me to identify these triggers so that I could avoid them and space out the crises.

In my case, the pain lasts 48 hours after it starts. The onset is slow and progresses until it becomes very annoying. As the hours pass, other symptoms are associated with it, such as hypersensitivity to light (with even TV or cell phone light bothering me) and nausea.

Some of the tricks that work for me are resting in a dark and quiet place with a comfortable temperature and drinking a strong black coffee with one or two aspirins. I usually repeat this treatment every 8 hours, sometimes without the coffee depending on how intense the pain is.

After 48 hours, I may be left with some hypersensitivity in the scalp; however, it is a self-limiting feeling that improves quickly.

3. Neck Pain

The most common cause of neck pain is the contracture of the spinal muscles. When this contracture involves the muscles on both sides of the neck, making mobilization difficult, it is called torticollis.

Poor posture can change the natural position of the vertebrae, causing discomfort, dizziness, and sometimes pain in the arms.

Neck pain rarely has anything to do with serious pathology. Most commonly, these are conditions that can be easily resolved.

Treatment

Painkillers, especially Naproxen, are a good choice for neck pain. Ibuprofen in doses between 600 and 800 mg also acts as a powerful anti-inflammatory that improves even torticollis. This is what I take when I have severe neck contractures:

- **Naproxen tablets 220 mg**- Dosage: 2 tablets every 6 hours for 5 days
- **Ibuprofen tablets 200mg** - Dosage for neck pain: 600 mg every 8 hours for 5 days

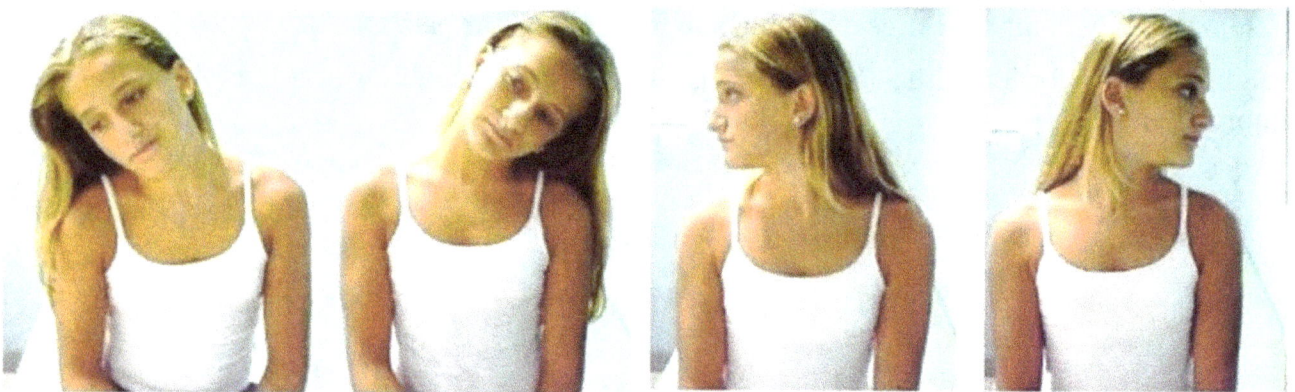

Ασκήσεις Αυχένος - Neck Exercises. Photo: Harry Gouvas "Neuroanatomy and Orthopaedic Neurology", 1988

Harrygouvas, Own work., CC BY-SA 3.0

Neck relaxation exercises, especially when working long hours in front of a computer screen, are important to avoid contracture. Every hour, you should move your neck to each side and make half-circles for two minutes. Every two hours, you should get out of your chair and walk around.

Working as an article writer, I often find myself in this situation. When talking to a friend who is an occupational physician, I was able gather some recommendations that I currently apply. My work chairis aligned with the computer screen, and I connected a keyboard to place it lower so that my arms are in a more ergonomic position.

When I finish work, I lie down by placing a pillow or towel roll right behind my neck. This relieves the tension on the muscles and helps them relax.

When Should I Worry?

If the neck pain is caused by a car accident or a hard impact on the head, it may be something more serious than a contracture since the neck suffers an injury known as **neck strain** or *whiplash*.

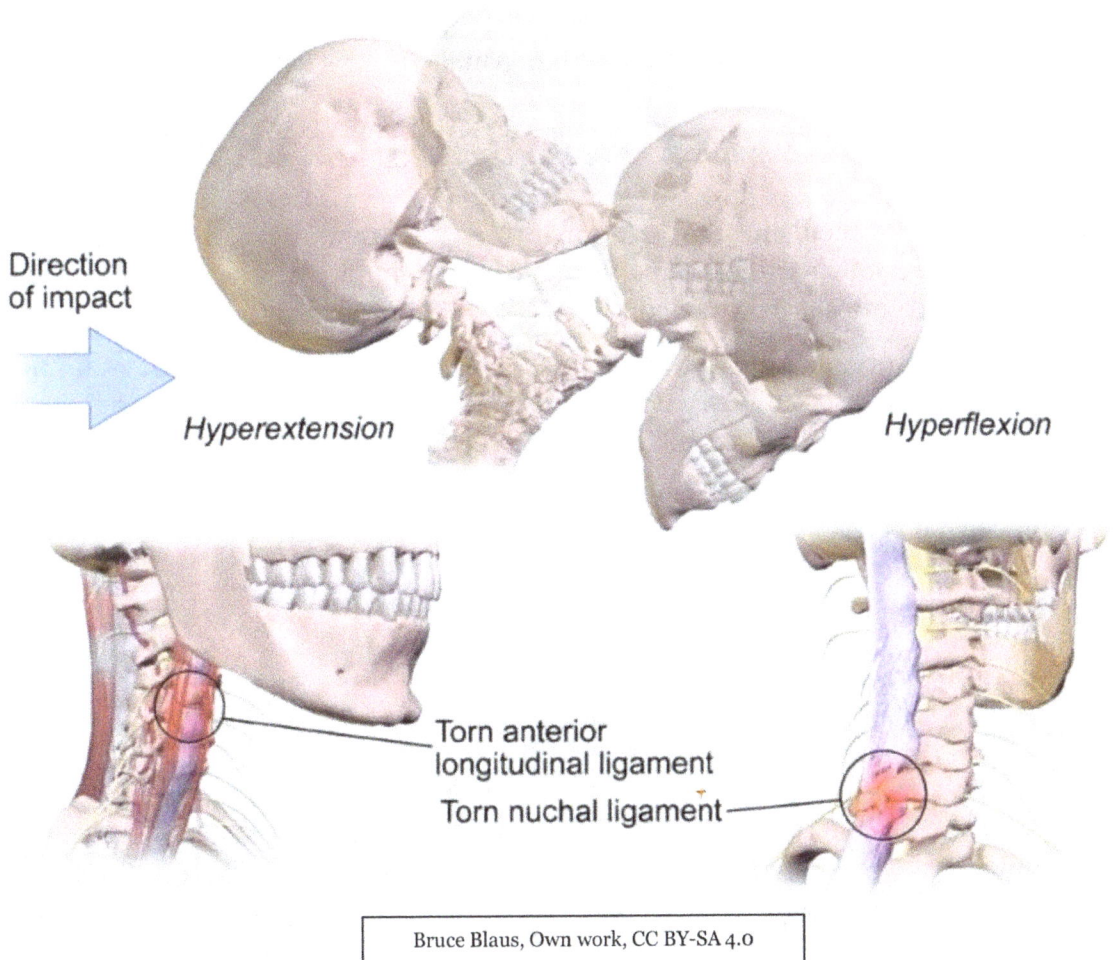

Bruce Blaus, Own work, CC BY-SA 4.0

Whiplash is a severe contraction of the muscles of the neck due to an abrupt deceleration that causes the head to rebound rapidly, stretching and contracting the muscles and ligaments of the neck very quickly.

With this condition, it is important to seek help since it is necessary to perform a neck x-ray and a magnetic resonance imaging (MRI) to observe the degree of modification of the spine and the indemnity of the vertebrae and ligaments.

It is important to seek help since it is necessary to perform a neck x-ray and a magnetic resonance imaging (MRI) to observe the degree of modification of the spine and the indemnity of the vertebrae and ligaments.

When the injury is not severe, treatment is based on analgesic therapy and physical rehabilitation, with specific exercises for each muscle group planned by a physiotherapist.

For more serious injuries, treatment will depend on the damage. Sometimes the treatment is medical, with placement of a hard cervical collar and observation, and other times the treatment is surgical.

Although some specialists still indicate the use of the cervical collar, that depends on the degree of injury, the patient's range of motion, and, ultimately, the treating physician.

In the hospital where I work, the protocol in cases of neck strain and sprain is early initiation of physical therapy, to preserve muscle strength. When the neck rests on the cervical collar, the muscles often become weakened and physical therapy takes longer than usual.

4. Eyes and Appendages of the Eye

Ophthalmology is the field of medicine that deals with diseases of the eyes and their appendages. Although I never interacted much with that service, in my hospital, we did transplants and organ procurement, so in those surgeries, we coincided.

I worked in the abdominal organs, and they did the corneal surgery. I have always found this an interesting and important area, especially because of the importance of the eyes in our relationship with the environment.

In this section, I explain the most common eye problems that we see at the emergency room and ways to solve them at home, when possible.

Red Eye

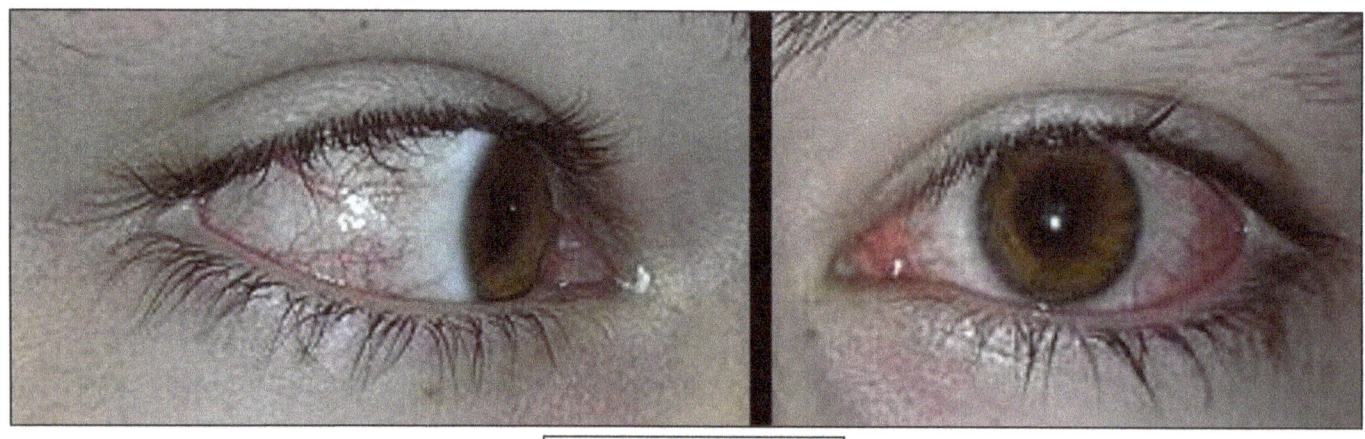

BrandonR, CC BY-SA 3.0

a) Causes

Dry eyes, **digital eye strain**, and **contact lenses** are common causes of red eye. Skin **allergies** are strongly associated with tearing and red eye. If you are a person suffering from rhinitis, dermatitis, and other allergies, it is very likely that contact with some substance or particle will irritate your eyes.

Environmental **pollution** in many cities also causes irritation of the ocular mucosa. In the summer, when there are extreme temperatures, forest fires fill the environment with **smoke**. This smoke can also cause eye discomfort.

Eye infections or **conjunctivitis** (pink eye) are a frequent cause of eye irritation associated with discharge, which can be transparent if is caused by a virus or purulent if caused by a bacteria. Conjunctivitis has other symptoms, such as itching and a gritty feeling inside the eye. One or both eyes could be affected.

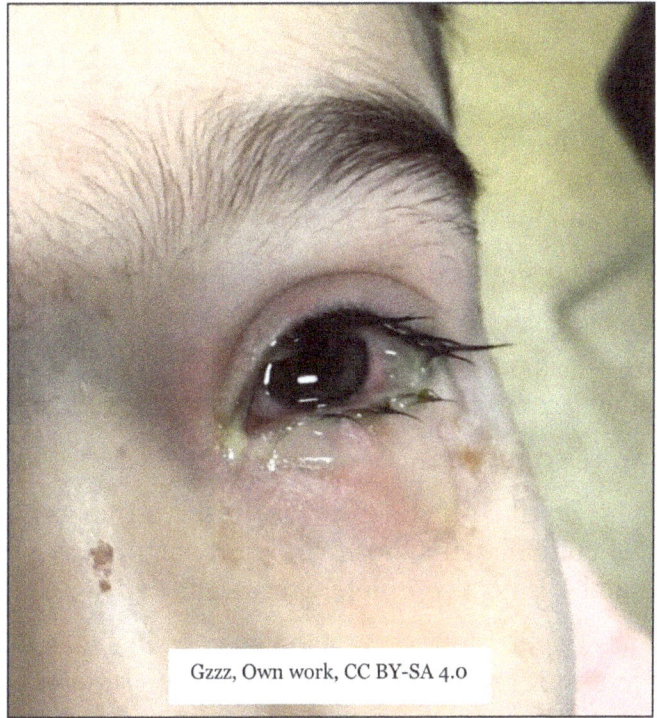

Gzzz, Own work, CC BY-SA 4.0

More serious conditions, such as increased intraocular pressure (**glaucoma**) or **corneal ulcer**, occur with red eye and are associated with pain.

Of these latter options, glaucoma is much more common, especially in the elderly.

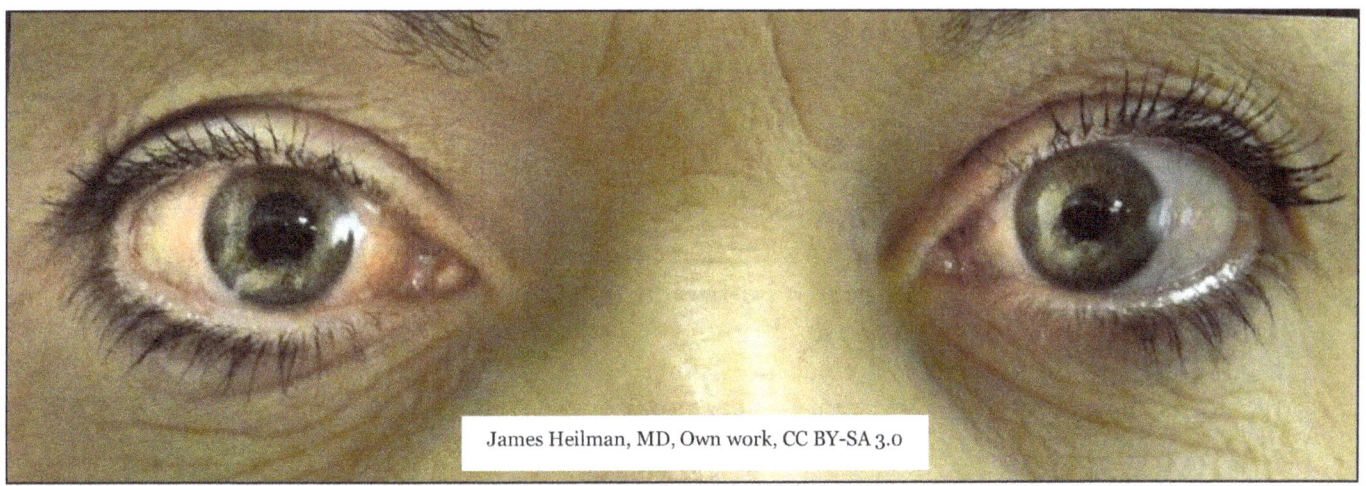

James Heilman, MD, Own work, CC BY-SA 3.0

In addition to red eye, glaucoma can present with eye pain and progressive loss of field vision. The easiest way to measure eye pressure is with a special device used by ophthalmologists and optometrists called a tonometer.

If you are diagnosed with glaucoma, it may be a good idea to keep a tonometer at home since increased intraocular pressure must be medicated because it can lead to permanent blindness.

It is not a cheap device because it is very specialized; however, in an exceptional state in which asking for help is not an option, it is the only way to know the intraocular pressure.

b) Treatment

In order to establish an appropriate treatment for red eye, we must know what is causing it. Irritation from allergies and exposure to smoke and other pollutants is self-limiting. Eye drops containing moisturizers relieve this symptom for these conditions.

The drops that we find over the counter are Hypo Tears, Soothe Long Lasting, and Eye Relief, among others. You can use two drops in each eye every six hours.

As for red eye due to dryness, it is better to use eye ointments or gels, especially at night, as they are more durable. Then you can do a combined treatment and use drops during the day and gel to sleep.

Some gels that are found over the counter are GenTeal Severe Dry Eye and Refresh Celluvisc.

Antibiotic eye drops are rarely used. In fact, these are reserved for patients with weakened immune systems. The vast majority of conjunctivitis, both viral and bacterial, is self-limiting. Therefore, within 72 hours, the condition should be almost completely resolved.

Remember that any substance applied to the eye can cause serious damage. The sclera and cornea are very delicate tissues, so unless they are products made by a laboratory. *I DO NOT ADVISE NATURAL TREATMENT IN THESE CASES.*

The use of chamomile and other infusions can harm rather than help. Despite being a good anti-inflammatory, chamomile is very astringent, meaning that it dries out the area where it is applied. It can therefore make the situation of the diseased eye worse.

To clean eye secretions, you can use a cotton wool with sterile saline solution or dip it in your eye drops. In the case of infection, try not to wash inside the eye with running water.

c) When Should I Worry?

- When **eye pain** or **partial vision loss** are associated
- If the **infection does not improve** after five days and the amount of discharge increases
- When there is continuous **blurred vision** and mild eye pain, there may be an ulcer on the cornea. To see it, you only have to light up the eye laterally and look at the membrane above the pupil. That membrane should be clear and smooth.
  Any abnormality can be an ulcer that requires specialized treatment.

Cataracts

The opacification of the lens of the eye is called a cataract. This condition usually develops slowly and is related to aging, although there are other causes.

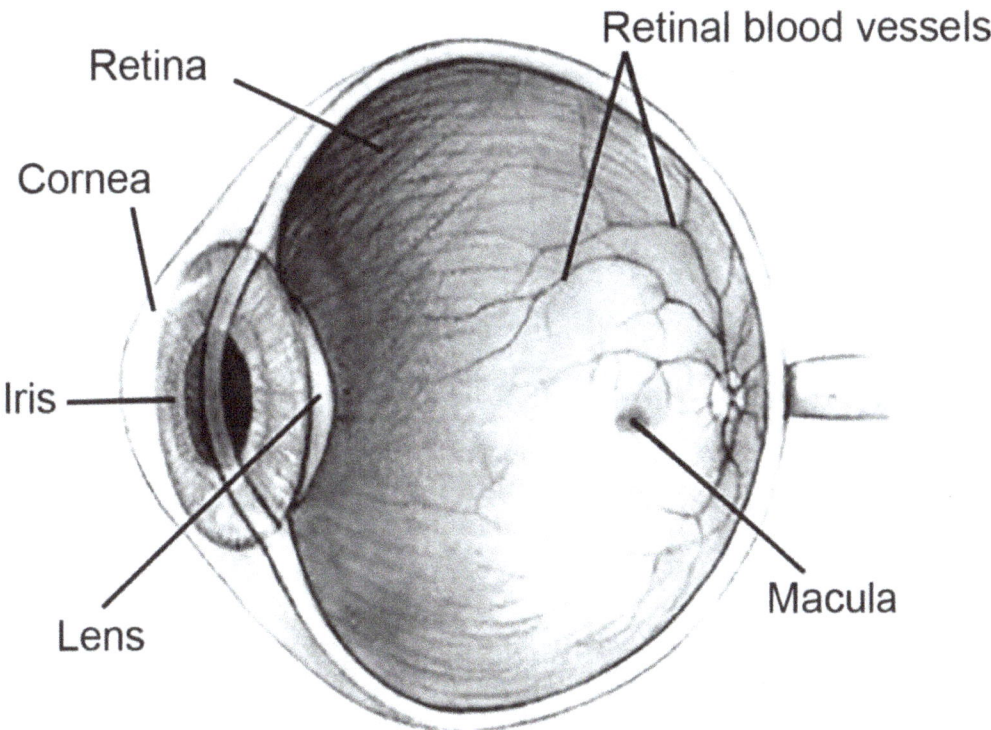

The main problem with this opacity is that it diminishes the quality of vision, causing blurred or double vision. It also intensifies the brightness that enters the eye, temporarily blinding the person and making it difficult to perform activities such as driving at night.

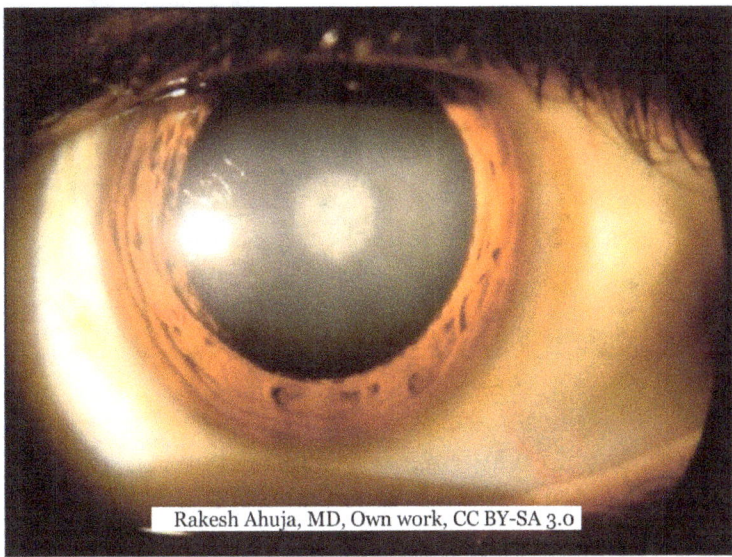

Rakesh Ahuja, MD, Own work, CC BY-SA 3.0

Some habits, such as smoking and drinking alcohol, have been linked to the development of cataracts. So have chronic diseases such as diabetes or the use of corticosteroid treatments.

The diagnosis is made on the basis of the physical examination by shining a light on the front of the eye so that light enters through the cornea.

In an eye without a cataract, the light should pass to the bottom of the globe.

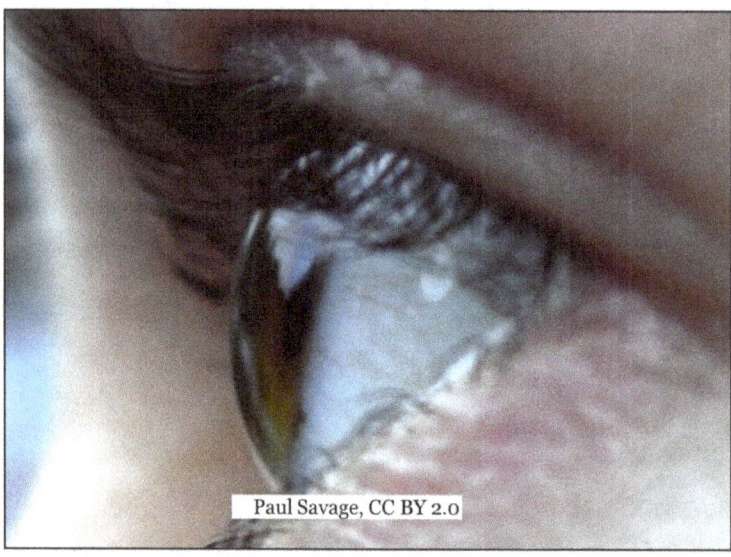
Paul Savage, CC BY 2.0

In an eye with a cataract, the light stops when it finds the opacity of the lens, which then becomes visible.

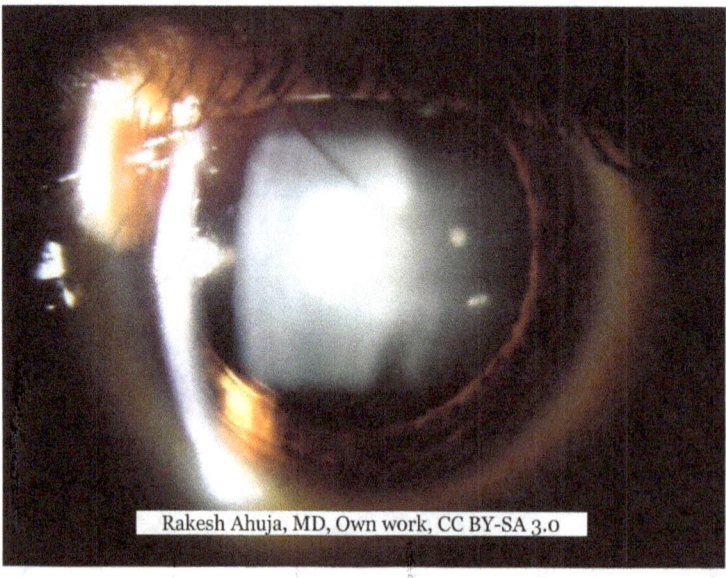
Rakesh Ahuja, MD, Own work, CC BY-SA 3.0

Cataract gold standard treatment is surgery; however, this is not the first treatment option in all cases. When the patient hasn't undergone surgery, he should have periodic appointments with his ophthalmologist and evaluate his visual capacity to see that it has not diminished.

It is always necessary to assess how advanced the condition is and the state of the patient before subjecting him or her to surgery, no matter how simple it may be. The cataract can lead to a state of temporary blindness that is reversed when the opaque lenses are removed.

a) Is There Any Way to Prevent the Development of Cataracts?

There is evidence that following some good habits can prevent and delay the onset of cataracts. Cigarettes and alcohol are directly related to their development, and their discontinuation decreases the possibility of this condition.

Although there is no strong evidence, a diet rich in green vegetables with natural antioxidants has been shown to be beneficial for eye health in general and specifically for slowing down cataract formation.

The use of sunglasses with adequate protection against ultraviolet rays makes it possible to reduce the exposure of the ocular components to solar radiation and to serve as a preventive tool.

Finally, it is important not to use eye drops indiscriminately, as some are composed of corticosteroids that cause chronic and sustained cell damage, leading to lens damage.

b) Do I Have Any Other Treatment Options?

Since 2017 there has been evidence that antioxidant N-acetyl carnosine (NAC) drops can stop and even reverse the development of cataracts. Currently the scientific evidence is not solid, but there are testimonials from patients who have seen improvement with the application of this product.

I do recommend it since some of my patients have seen improve of cataracts symptoms while using it.

Eye Pain

Eye pain is a fairly common and not usually an alarming symptom. However, there are some serious conditions in which pain is the main symptom.

The causes of this pain are varied, and some of these commonly occur and do not represent major complications, such as the presence of foreign bodies, infections, contact lens irritation, blepharitis or inflammation of the eyelids, and sties.

In all of these conditions, pain appears as one more symptom, which improves completely when the infection is treated or the foreign body is removed.

One eye pain I'm very familiar with is dengue fever. About ten years ago, there was an epidemic of that disease in my country. The topic of conversation when you met anyone was whether they had dengue fever and, if so, what type (hemorrhagic or classic) and what symptoms they had.

Pain behind the eyes is a constant symptom that is part of the development of dengue fever. It's such intense pain that it bothers you to even move them a little bit sideways.

Although it lasts only a few days, it overwhelms you. I ended up being infected in the two epidemics in Venezuela. What luck!

When Should I Worry?

Eye pain that has no apparent cause should always be a cause for concern. Glaucoma, which is the increase in eye pressure, causes this type of pain. When associated with vision loss, you can make this diagnostic approach that represents an absolute emergency in which it is necessary to seek help since the patient may lose their vision permanently.

Migraine and sinusitis are diseases that are not typical of the eyes but are closely related and cause this symptom. I suffered from continuous migraines for a long time, and I can say that when eye pain is associated with headache, it is hopeless. It's very difficult to find relief.

My way of fighting it is by drinking black coffee and lying down in a very dark room with the right temperature. If the pain continues after 48 hours or after the migraine episode has passed, it is important to tell a specialist. It may not be an emergency that requires you to attend a care center, but it is good to have the advice of a professional.

Stye

A stye, or hordeolum, is a pimple along the line of the eyelashes. It is usually filled with pus, becomes very swollen, and can cause pain. It can be found on the outside of the eye or inside the eyelid.

Its location does not determine its aggressiveness. In fact, these types of injuries are quite benign.

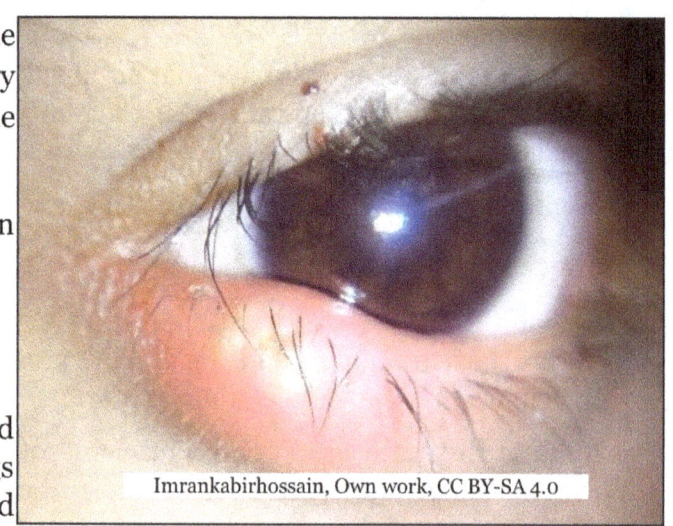
Imrankabirhossain, Own work, CC BY-SA 4.0

Treatment

Sties are self-limiting. They rarely get complicated and need to be drained. There are still some things we can do, however, to relieve the inflammation and speed up the healing process.

Taking an anti-inflammatory or pain reliever may help with the pain. Placing compresses with water or warm solution also improves inflammation.

In my country, it is said that heating a spoon and pressing it on the stye is the ultimate cure for this disease. Strangely enough, it works. The combination of pressure and heat on the injury improves the symptoms quite a lot.

However, I would exchange the spoon for a towel or cloth with hot water, even though the ladies from the rural parts of Venezuela will be disappointed with this replacement.

Blepharitis

Blepharitis is a fairly common condition involving infection and inflammation of the eyelids. This occurs because bacteria that normally inhabit the skin can invade any area that presents a small wound.

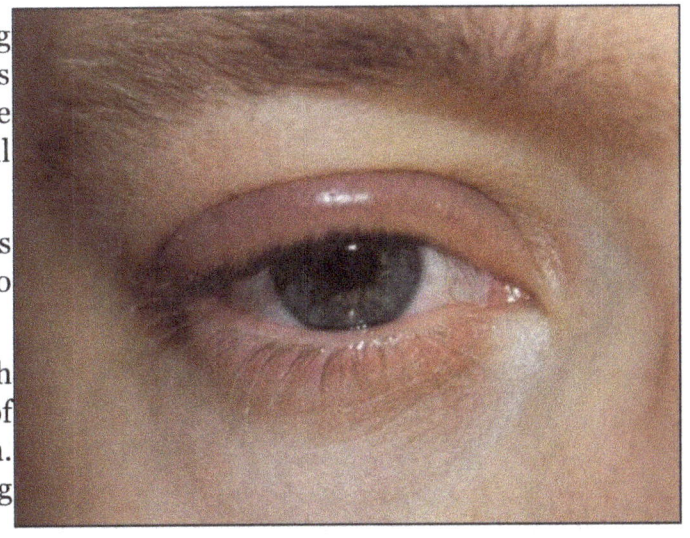

Vigorous scratching, skin irritation, or insect bites become gateways for these microorganisms to contaminate and start the process.

This infection is easily diagnosed through inspection of the eyelid. The classic signs of inflammation are red, hardened, and swollen skin. In addition, this skin has the peculiarity of flaking off like dandruff.

Blepharitis can be anterior (external) or posterior, just at the edge of the eyelash line and even inside, and is often associated with the processes of seborrheic dermatitis and dandruff.

Treatment

The treatment of blepharitis, at least in its early stages, does not include special medications. Proper eyelid hygiene with a moist towel is recommended.

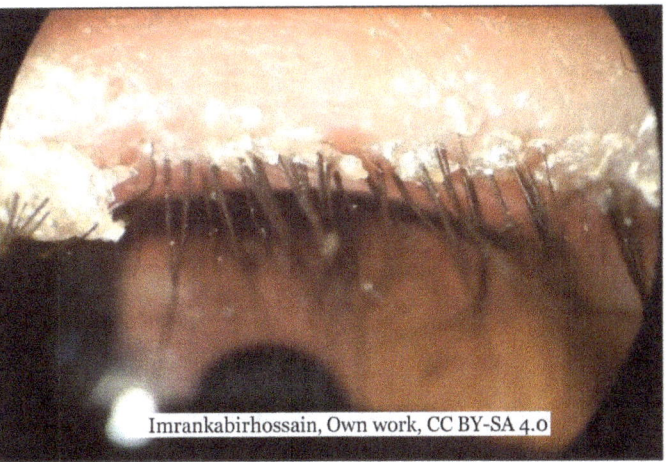

Imrankabirhossain, Own work, CC BY-SA 4.0

An ophthalmologist friend of mine always recommends using baby shampoo that does not irritate the eye mucosa to perform this cleaning, along with warm water, at least twice a day.

If flakes are observed, they should be removed; this can be done with a swab, softly and without pressing hard. In this type of infection, the eyelid becomes very sensitive because some glands may be clogged.

To help them discharge their contents, gently massage the entire eyelid for five minutes before cleaning. Blepharitis resolves in a few days if proper hygiene measures are taken.

Although in many places you will find information about the usefulness of chamomile in the eyes, either for making eye washes or as eye drops, this liquid is not recommended.

Chamomile is a natural astringent, meaning that it absorbs moisture. It is excellent for some skin therapies, but that effect on the eye makes it lose its lubrication and dry out, causing other problems.

RESPIRATORY SYSTEM

The respiratory system is an anatomical apparatus that consists of the airways and the lungs, and it allows the exchange of gases in the body, which is the exit of carbon dioxide and the entry of oxygen into the blood, allowing for the vitality of tissues and organs.

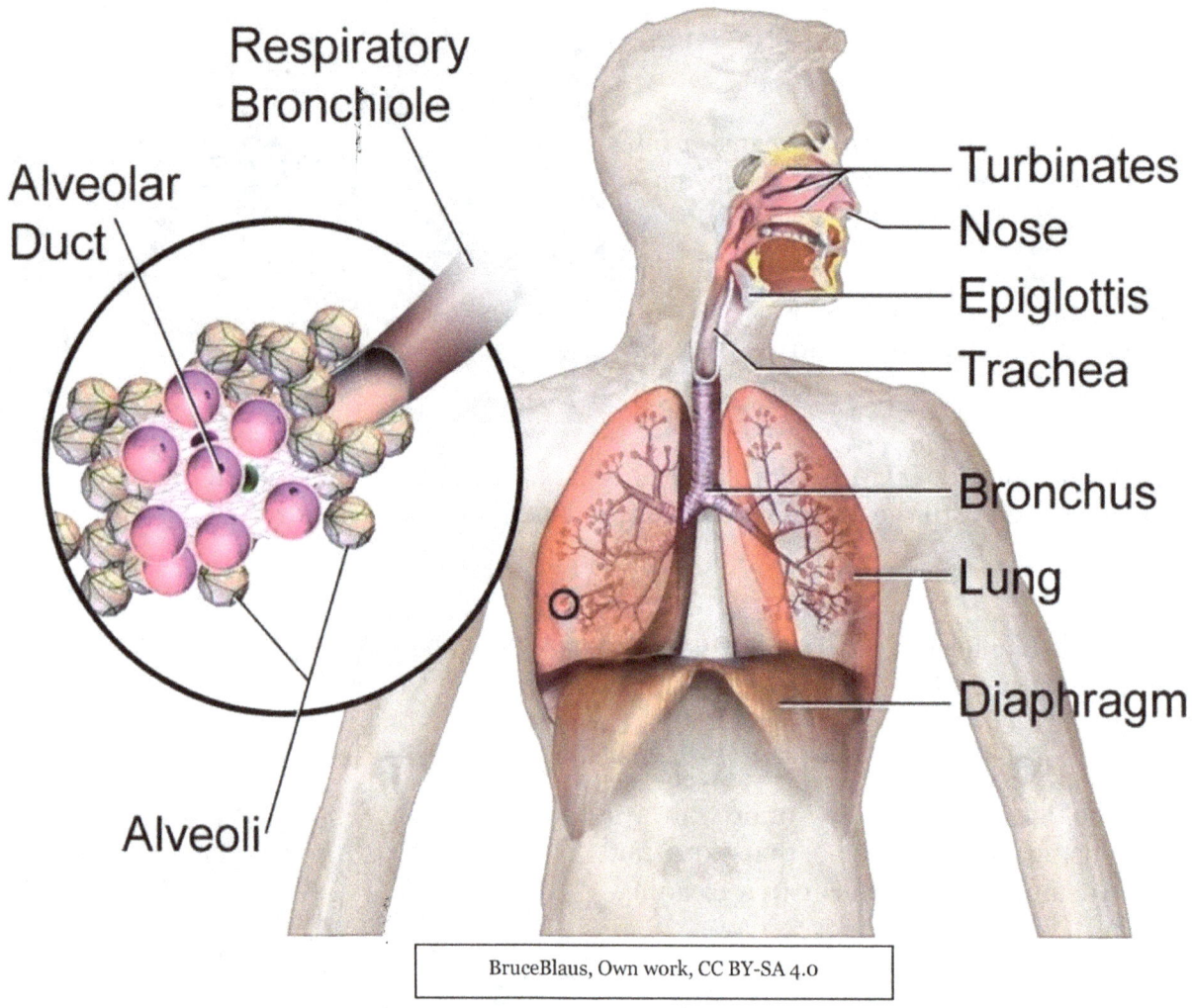

BruceBlaus, Own work, CC BY-SA 4.0

The breathing rate is the number of times a person breathes in a given amount of time. Normal is about twelve to twenty breaths in a minute. This is called **eupnea**. A person who breathes normally, at a rateof twelve breaths per minute and without any effort, is *eupneic*. From that number, we can classify the breath in:

- **Tachypnea:** more than 20 breaths in 1 minute
- **Bradipnea:** less than 12 breaths in a minute
- **Dyspnea:** breathing with effort or shortness of breath

Each of these respiratory types has specific causes that will be explained throughout this chapter.

1. Cough

Coughing is one of the main medical complaints and is included in 40% of the visits to pulmonologists. It is a reflex that is part of the body's defense system. It helps expel foreign materials, whether bacteria, dust, or another foreign body, from the airways.

Coughing is a very vague symptom that is associated with many causes. It is difficult to arrive at a specific diagnosis based on this data alone since no objective classifications have been defined to guide the different cases.

Coughs can be arbitrarily classified into acute and chronic. It is acute if it lasts less than three weeks, and chronic if it lasts longer than that. It can also be classified as dry or wet (productive), depending on whether it produces secretions or not.

Most Common Causes

Acute cough:

- Common cold virus
- Flu
- Allergies
- Bronchitis
- Dust or smoke inhalation

Chronic cough:

- Pneumonia
- Tuberculosis
- Chronic obstructive pulmonary disease (COPD)
- Lung cancer (not a constant symptom)
- Postnasal drip
- Gastroesophageal reflux disease (GERD)
- Side effect of some antihypertensive drugs

It is important to recognize non-respiratory causes since the cough will not go away until what is causing it is removed. Coughing caused by GERD usually occurs at night or after a large meal. It may be accompanied by vomiting and is associated with gastric symptoms.

For antihypertensive drugs, it's a matter of locating the start of the cough in the timeline and seeing if it coincides with the start of the medication.

My recommendation is that if you change your medications, always keep track of treatment initiation to monitor side effects and other symptoms.

Treatment

a) Alternative Medicine and Natural Treatments

Natural treatments to relieve coughs are based on improving the irritation of the airways. This is achieved through hydration, which allows the fluidization of secretions and the improvement of the inflammation of the larynx.

Honey is a powerful anti-inflammatory as well as helping to heal the irritated mucous membrane of the larynx by eliminating the unpleasant sensation of a scratchy throat. Mixing two teaspoons of honey with warm water or tea is helpful before going to sleep.

When coughing is associated with a sore throat, the mixture of honey and milk is fantastic; it is a therapy that has been used in my family for a long time. Honey can be consumed together with other medications since it does not cause any unfavorable effects, and its benefits are huge.

Ginger is also a natural anti-inflammatory that helps clear the airways. Its properties have been used since the beginning of Asian medicine for different diseases.

It can be consumed as tea, chewed directly, or prepared as candy with some sweetener, sugar, or honey.

Steam baths are excellent decongestants. They help moisten the airways and mobilize viscous secretions. This can be done once a day by heating water to a boil and breathing in the steam. To do this, lean over the container and place a towel over your head.

All my childhood, I was very allergic. Dust and cold caused me to have severe coughing spells that madeit difficult to breathe normally. I remember my mother would boil water with a few drops of eucalyptusoil in a pot, and I would breathe in that steam until there was no more left. It was comforting and helpedme rest.

Remember that steam can burn the skin. It is important not to stand too close to it, and if there is discomfort on the skin, step away and wait 30 seconds to one minute before continuing.

Saltwater gargle is a good choice for very productive coughs as it helps to expel secretions and decrease the amount of mucus. This combination is especially good for post-nasal drip. To prepare the gargle, mix a 1/2 teaspoon of salt with half a cup of warm water. It can be repeated during the day as many times as necessary.

b) OTC Cough Medicine

There are two types of cough treatments: **antitussives** and **expectorants**. Antitussives serve to stop the cough reflex, while expectorants thin out secretions to make them easier to cough up.

The best-known cough suppressant is *Dextromethorphan*. It is found in many types of syrups, along with other compounds. Some brands are Triaminic Cold and Cough, Robitussin Cough, and Vicks 44 Cough and Cold.

As for expectorants, those that are obtained over the counter are the ones that contain *Guaifenesin* (Mucinex, Robitussin Chest Congestion).

There are syrups and tablets that combine two ingredients, such as Robitussin DM. Otherwise these active ingredients can be found individually in various types of treatments, combined with antihistamines and anti-inflammatories, such as in cold medicines.

If the only symptom you have is a cough, you should look for specific medications for this. Treatments that combine antihistamines can be counterproductive because that type of medicine dries out the lining of the throat and dries out the mucus, which can further irritate the airways and trigger your cough reflex.

When Should I Worry?

- If you have difficulty breathing and swallowing that doesn't get better in eight hours.
- If the cough persists for more than three weeks.
- When weight loss and night sweats are associated as these may be due to tuberculosis, which isa very contagious infection.
- If you notice blood mixed with phlegm.

It is important to know that when you make a lot of effort to cough, some blood may come out of the mucosa, and it has nothing to do with an infection or other serious pathology. Blood mixed with phlegm and bright red blood after coughing are warning signs.

What Does Expectoration Mean?

Sputum, or phlegm, is only a defense response of the body to a pathogen or allergen. By observing the mucus, we can guide the diagnosis. A fluid and transparent phlegm is from an allergic process where there is irritation of the airway and mucus is formed to protect it.

Green or grayish mucus, sometimes with a strange smell, guides us to the presence of bacteria, such asin pneumonia. Sometimes it looks more purulent than others, but it is always oriented to the same diagnosis. Often this type of purulent sputum must be microbiologically cultured to find out which bacteria it is and which antibiotics it is susceptible to. When phlegm is accompanied by blood, it can be very shocking and cause concern. In these cases, we should try to evaluate the whole scene before thinking about a possible diagnosis.

If the patient has been coughing for many hours or days or has had coughing fits in which he or she has exerted himself or herself, the blood may be due to irritation or rupture of small vessels or the mucous membrane of the airway. However, if the blood is bright red or contains clots, it is a sign of damage to the bronchial tubes or to the lungs. These damages can be a tumor that is inside the bronchus and is bleeding, active tuberculosis that is excavating the lung, or lung cancer.

1. Ear, Nose, and Throat

Otolaryngology is the branch of medicine that studies the ears, nose and throat. Diseases of these three organs are very common. We have all had a sore throat or earache, and many of us have had nosebleeds, so it is a fairly familiar topic in which I seek only to clarify some points and supplement with tips that may be useful for solving problems when it is not possible to ask for specialized help.

Ear

The ear is the organ of hearing. It has an external and an internal component. The external is formed by the auricle or pinna and the external ear opening. The internal ear canal is a tunnel that connects the pinna with a set of small bones that vibrate so that we can identify sounds.

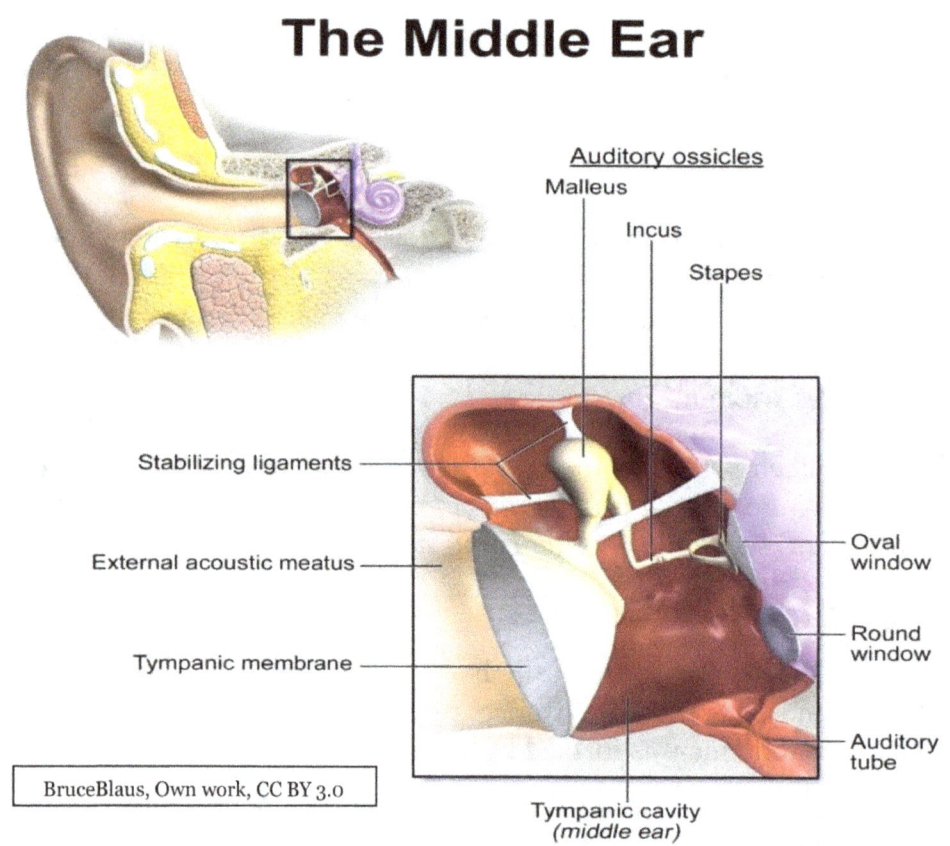

The skin of this tunnel is delicate, and about one inch away is a membrane that separates the ear canal into the outer and middle, where the bones are located. Damage to the membrane can cause serious damage, such as contamination of the middle ear canal and hearing loss.

a) Cleaning the Ear Canal: Removing Foreign Bodies and Earwax Plugs

Earwax is a fatty, semi-solid product secreted by ear cells that serves as protection against damage and microorganisms that can enter the ear canal. There is always the question of how to clean the ear canal safely, especially if there is an impaction of wax that causes pain and discharge.

Q-tips are not recommended for cleaning the ear, basically because many people do not use them properly. To clean with the Q-tips, you should make circular movements and push outward, not toward the eardrum. Accidents occur when you try to push the swab in too far or when you clean the wax excessively. Remember that wax is a protection against infection and micro-particles. Trying to remove it completely leaves the ear susceptible to pathogens.

When I worked in Brazil, I had many patients with wax impacts or foreign bodies inside the ear canal. The most common were insects and paper, but in children and very old patients, you can find any kind of object, even beans and rice.

Some people use paper to prevent insects from getting into their ears, and the debris builds up inside, mixing with earwax and forming a very thick blockage that is difficult to remove. Sometimes the person is not sure they have an object in their ear.

When the patient comes in with ear discomfort, difficulty hearing in one ear and a feeling of blockage or slight pressure, simply shine a flashlight into the ear canal to see if there is a foreign body inside.

Once I identified the object, I used to perform a very effective and secure technique that never fails to remove any foreign body inside the ear.

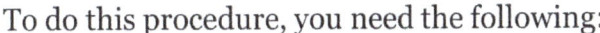
Anand2202, Own work, CC BY-SA 4.0

To do this procedure, you need the following:

- 1 feeding tube or 1 butterfly syringe
- 1 syringe of 20cc or larger
- Saline solution
- Optional: earwax removal drops

The patient should be lying or sitting down but not standing up, as ear canal irrigation may cause dizziness. To lessen this effect, you can heat the salt solution a little.

Procedure:

1. Connect the scalp or feeding catheter to the 20cc syringe. If you have a scalp, you must cut the needle so as to leave only the plastic tube.

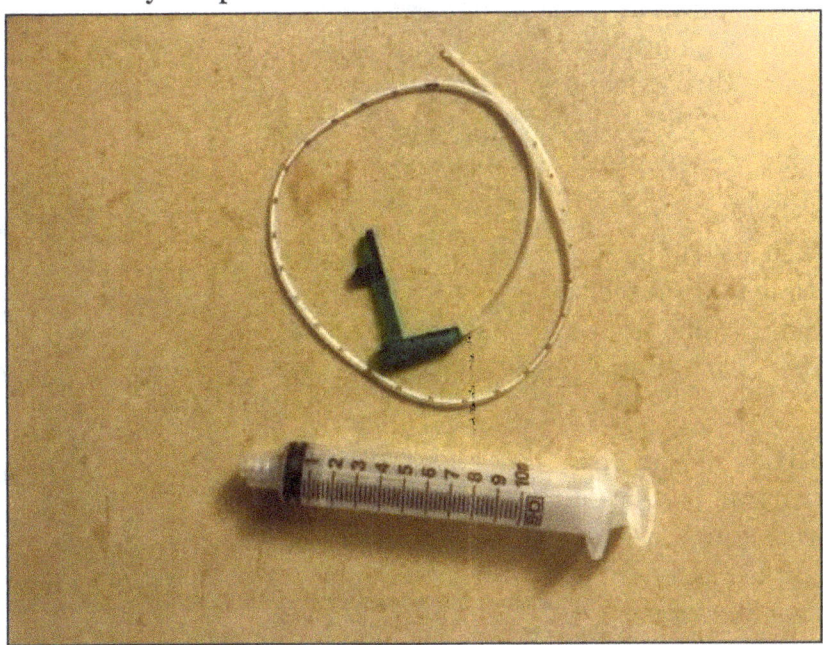

2. Fill the syringe up to 20 or 30cc, depending on the capacity of the one you have.

3. Insert the tube into your ear canal about 0.5 inches and start irrigating firmly but not too quickly.

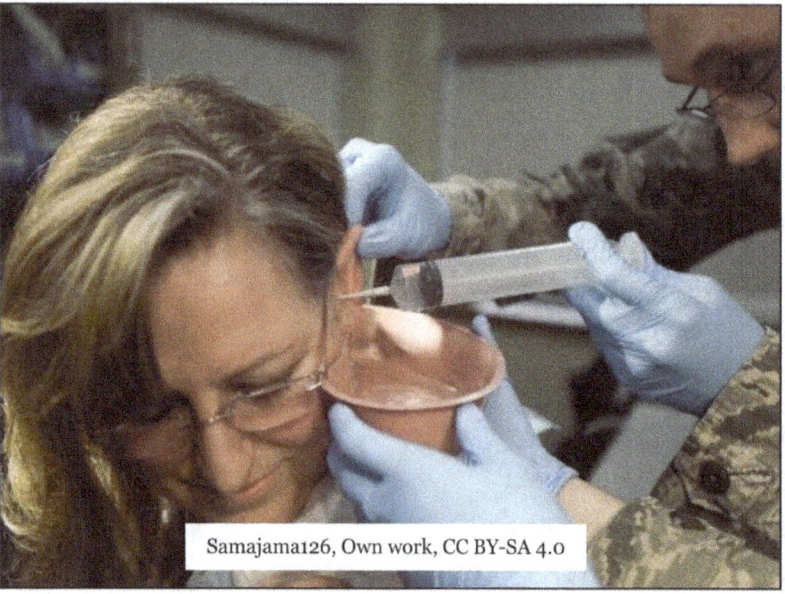
Samajama126, Own work, CC BY-SA 4.0

Under the patient's ear, you can place a bedding center or a container to prevent them from getting wet. You can repeat the procedure, but I don't think you'll have to. All of the contents that were blocking the ear will come out without you having to do anything else.

If you find that the impacted earwax is too thick or large, you can apply a few drops of earwax remover first, which will help soften it.

b) Earache

Ear pain is a fairly common symptom that can occur for reasons that have nothing to do with the ear. Colds, sore throats, sinus infections, dental issues like cavities, and temporomandibular joint problems are some of the causes of earache.

Even some sounds, such as rubbing or whistling, can be due to dental problems, as happened to a friend who stopped hearing a noise in her ear after her orthodontic treatment.

Ear infection, or **otitis,** is the main cause of pain and can occur for various reasons, such as earwax plug; a virus; stagnant water in a pool, at the beach, or in a bathtub; and bacterial infections.

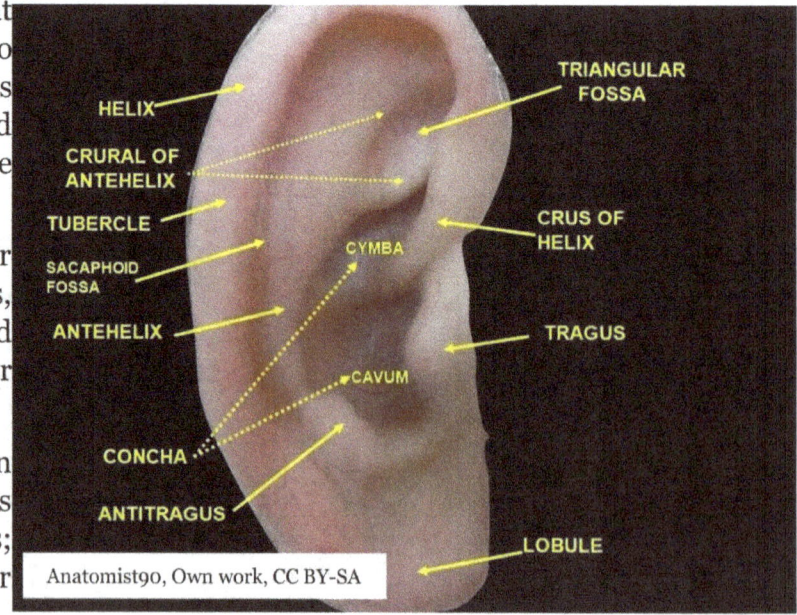
Anatomist90, Own work, CC BY-SA

A simple way to diagnose it without using expensive instruments is to evaluate the auricular pavilion for redness in the external auditory canal.

Pull the earlobe down for a few seconds and see if it causes discomfort. Pressing the tragus firmly also increases the pressure on the eardrum, causing pain. Usually, the agents that cause otitis are viral and the process is self-limiting.

The treatment is symptomatic, and analgesics such as NSAIDs are indicated for three days to improve the pain.

For pain after swimming, the so-called **swimmer's ear**, the application of drops is indicated to help dry out the remaining water and humidity in the ear canal, as well as analgesics. The difference in **pressure** can cause severe pain in one or both ears. You may have felt this on a plane trip, in an elevator, or on any trip to a place where the pressure changes dramatically.

The problem in these cases is that the eardrum, which is the membrane that separates the external part of the ear from the internal part, does not balance the internal pressure with the external pressure fast enough, generating a lot of pain.

One of the techniques recommended by a flight attendant was chewing gum. Trying to blow with a blocked nose can also achieve the necessary pressure, but this technique can generate so much pressure that it can perforate the eardrum, so I avoid it. Gum always produces excellent results.

It is rare for an adult otitis process to become complicated to the point of requiring antibiotics. However, if after four days with anti-inflammatory treatment the symptoms continue or worsen, or discharge is added through the ear, antibiotic treatment should be started, and you should notify the specialist so that he or she can take your case into account.

The antibiotic of choice is Amoxicillin 250 mg every 8 hours for 7 days. If you are allergic to penicillin, you can take Ciprofloxacin 500 mg every 12 hours for 10 days.

c) Tinnitus

If you've ever been to a concert or a nightclub with loud music for a long time, I'm sure you know what tinnitus is. The term tinnitus refers to the sensation of hearing a buzzing or whistling in the ear that can be continuous or intermittent, steady or pulsating. It is a fairly common cause of consultation.

It is triggered by a number of causes, including exposure to loud sounds either from work (construction, carpentry) or fun, blockage of the ear canal by a foreign body, use of some drugs like aspirin and some antidepressants, an early symptom of hearing loss, or cervical, dental, and temporomandibular joint problems.

Tinnitus can be a symptom of a disease such as high blood pressure or hyperthyroidism. In this case, the sound is pulsating because what is heard is the sound of blood passing through the arteries.

In the clinical evaluation, the doctor can hear the noise with the stethoscope; that is why it is known as objective tinnitus.

Once therapy is given for the underlying disease, the sound decreases or stops. In many cases, tinnitus is related to a neurological hearing problem; however, it has no major health impact. It has no specific treatment beyond relaxation techniques.

When the trigger is the use of a drug or exposure to loud sounds, the tinnitus should stop when the cause is removed. Special hearing aids are recommended for people who work in noisy environments.

d) Hearing Loss

Hearing loss is the inability to hear sounds that everyone normally hears. Although hearing impairment and hearing loss are used interchangeably, the truth is that the former refers to the difficulty of hearing but not to the impossibility.

Age is the most common cause of progressive hearing loss. From the age of 65 onward, about half of all people have some degree of hearing impairment, and this number increases with age.

The main consequences of hearing loss and hearing impairment are to social and work relationships, which can lead to anxiety and depression. In addition, there is a relationship between hearing loss and accidental falls.

Although hearing difficulty occurs in the elderly, steps can be taken to avoid it or slow it down. There are professions that expose people to developing hearing loss, including construction, carpentry, nightclub clerks, and MRI technicians.

The relationship between aircrew members and hearing loss has also been studied both because of the noise and because of the continuous pressure changes to which they are exposed.

Prevention

- Avoid continuous exposure to loud noise.
- If working in a noisy environment, try to use safety headphones.
- See a hearing specialist if you have symptoms of difficulty hearing so that the level of hearing can be determined and a device can be recommended to improve it.

Nose

a) Nosebleeds

Nosebleeds have many causes. It is common to see this in very dry climates, whether they are hot or cold, because the nasal mucosa gets dry and is very sensitive to changes in humidity. It can also be due to a traumatic event or changes in blood pressure.

In the ER, I have seen patients come in with heavy nosebleeds. Many people recommend putting your head back; in fact, you see it a lot on TV and movies. But this is not a good recommendation.

The blood that comes out of the nose comes from the front of the mucosa; by putting the head back, we swallow it, which can cause stomach upset.

It is ideal to lean forward and squeeze your nostrils for about ten seconds while you breathe through your mouth. The fingers are placed a little higher than the nostrils, without hurting the septum.

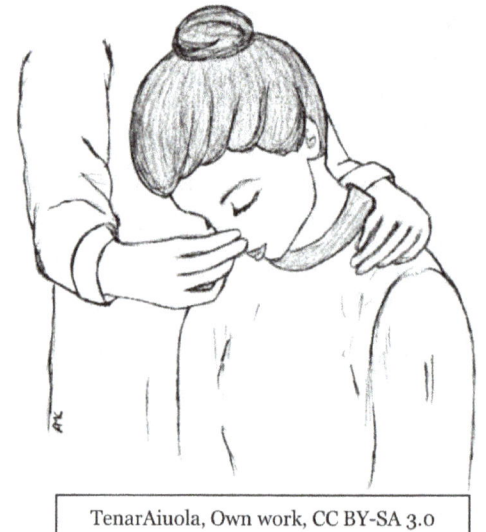

TenarAiuola, Own work, CC BY-SA 3.0

Putting ice on the top of your nose, between the eyes, is also good advice. I never recommend inserting paper or cotton into the nostrils. If something is introduced, I would choose to use gauze since it does not leave any remains inside the orifices.

b) Foreign Body in the Nose

The nose and ears are places where foreign bodies can commonly get stuck. In children and patients with dementia, this is more likely to occur; however, we must be vigilant as it is a situation that can occur at any time to anyone. If a foreign body is left in one of these holes and time passes, an infection could develop that may bring other complications.

Objects stuck in the nose are sometimes visible and can even be picked out with fingers or tweezers. The procedure to remove it must be done with outward movements, otherwise the object will be introduced further and may get stuck in the back of the nose, where it is not possible to remove it without specialized assistance.

If the object is visible inside the nose, you can try to remove it by covering the opposite side and asking the person to blow hard until it comes out. This procedure should be repeated until the foreign body comes out.

This option is very useful and one I recommend the most since it does not damage the mucosa and it is impossible for the object to get stuck in the back of the nose.

In the event that the object is badly stuck and does not come out by the above methods, a homemade device for extraction can be tried.

The original instrument used by ENT doctors is a surgical hook that you can build with a paper clip or with a wire that is not very rigid. In the picture to the right, you can see what the hook remover looks like.

Sarindam7, Own work, CC BY-SA 4.0

You're going to make a paper clip that has the same effect as the original instrument.

This instrument is gently inserted through the nostril where the foreign body is located and is then attached to the paper clip. All the movements must be very smooth and always trying to pull out. Remember that this mucosa is fragile and can bleed, but a little bit of blood is not something to worry about.

Once the foreign body is out, it should be checked for completeness. A spray such as Afrin, which contains a substance that constricts blood vessels and prevents bleeding, can be applied to the nostril.

The danger triangle of the face is an anatomical area described as the triangle formed between the outer edges of the mouth and the nasal septum. It includes the upper maxilla and the nose.

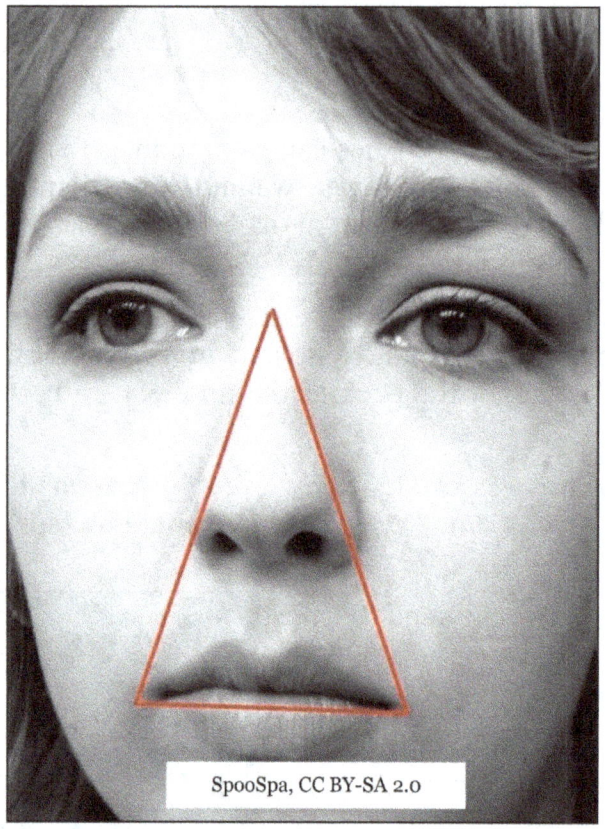
SpooSpa, CC BY-SA 2.0

It is called this because of the danger that an infection in this area can develop a serious consequence in the brain, such as a brain abscess or meningitis. This is possible because the circulation in this area is connected directly to the brain. Although it is not the most common, it is important to know that it can occur and that any type of infection involving the triangle should be treated promptly.

Throat

Sore Throat

A sore throat is a very common complaint. It is the inflammation of the upper airway, and it can be divided into three types depending on its location: tonsillitis, pharyngitis, and laryngitis.

It can be caused by viral and bacterial infections and has general symptoms, such as dryness, burning, itching, pain, irritation, and tenderness when swallowing.

Tonsillitis and pharyngitis do not present symptoms of voice loss, but the larynx is one of the structures involved in the process of creating sound, so its inflammation does show these symptoms.

Viral and bacterial infections of the tonsils cause different signs and symptoms. In viral infections, thereis redness of the pharynx and swelling of the tonsils, with general malaise and headache.
In the case of the bacterial infections, the disease is more obvious, presenting with high fever, pain, redness of the tonsils, and white spots on its surface that are plaques of pus.

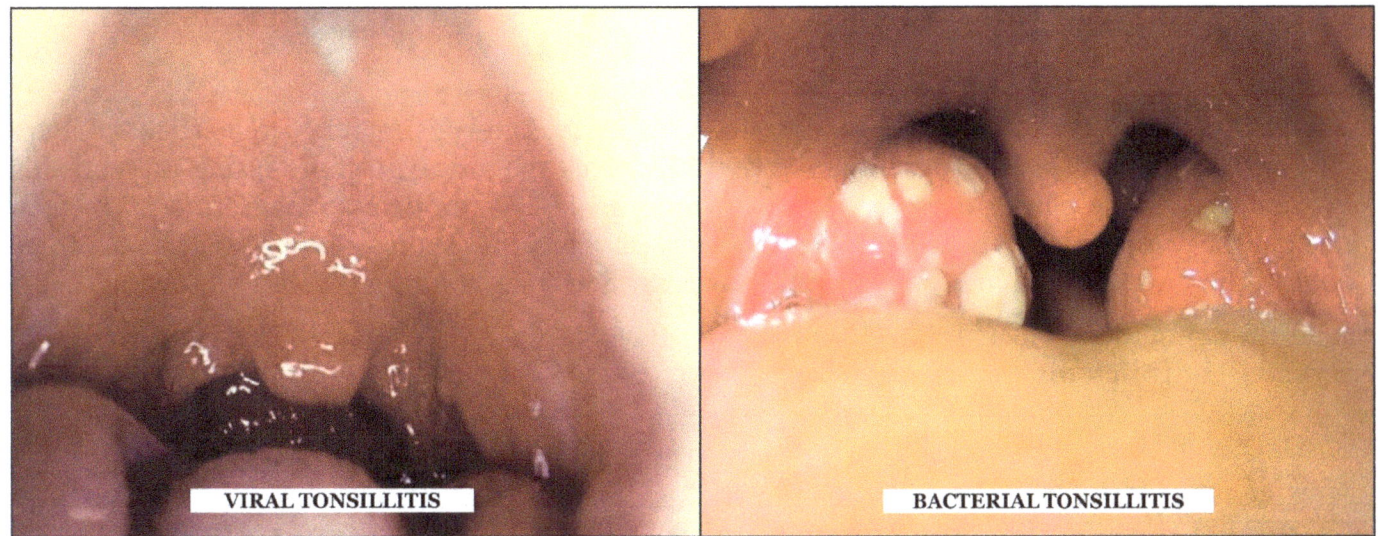

Treatment

There are many natural remedies for sore throats. My favorite is to drink warm milk with one tablespoon of honey. Honey is a powerful anti-inflammatory, and milk has relaxing properties. Milk can also be replaced by an infusion. Saltwater gargle and water with hydrogen peroxide gargle also work very well, but the latter can have an impact on tooth enamel.

Ginger is an excellent anti-inflammatory and antiseptic that has always been used for various ailments. Nowadays it is fashionable to take ginger shots. Ginger tea and candy can be made at home and are very helpful and widely used. Ginger chews can be bought anywhere for sore throats or gastrointestinal discomfort.

Chewable Crystallized Ginger

Ingredients:
- 1 pound of fresh ginger
- 1 ½ cups of honey
- 1 ½ cups of filtered water.

Preparation:

Peel and slice the ginger root. Put water and honey in a pot until it boils, and place the ginger over low heat until it is tender, about 30 minutes. Turn off the heat and let it cool. Pour through a strainer until all extra syrup falls off the ginger pieces. Set leftover pieces on wax paper to dry and crystallize for about 12 hours. During episodes of burning and scratching, I prefer to stay away from cold places or exposure to air conditioning.

When white plaques are seen on irritated tonsils, the infection is generated by bacteria, and you should receive antibiotics. One of the best options is Cephalexin 500 mg every 12 hours for 10 days.

Symptoms improve rapidly around the fourth day of treatment, but you should complete the ten-day course of antibiotics.

2. Airway Obstruction

Airway obstruction is very common, even if we don't realize it. Some obstructions are partial and don't lead to any complications. However, others completely block the airway, compromising the patient's ventilation. An airway blockage can occur at any time, so be aware of the maneuvers used to help yourself or the person who is choking. When a person is choking, they should get the attention of others by holding their neck in both hands. This is the universal chocking sign.

Usually, the object that is blocking the airway is expelled with coughing. If it doesn't come out, you can perform the **Heimlich maneuver**.

Heimlich Maneuver

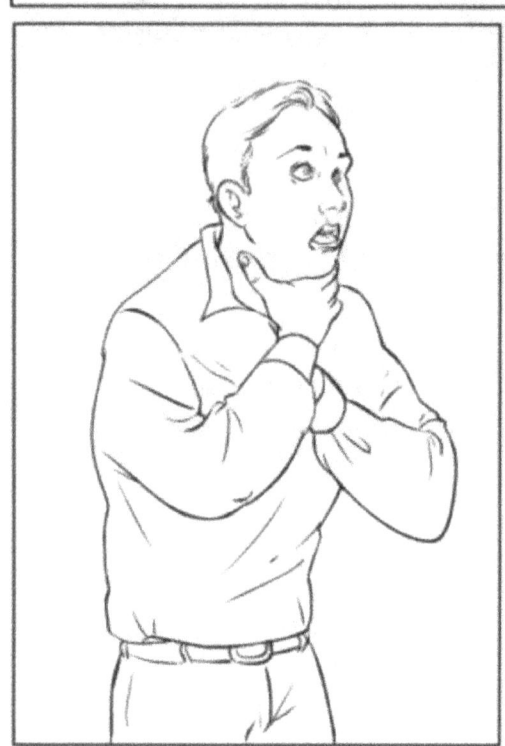
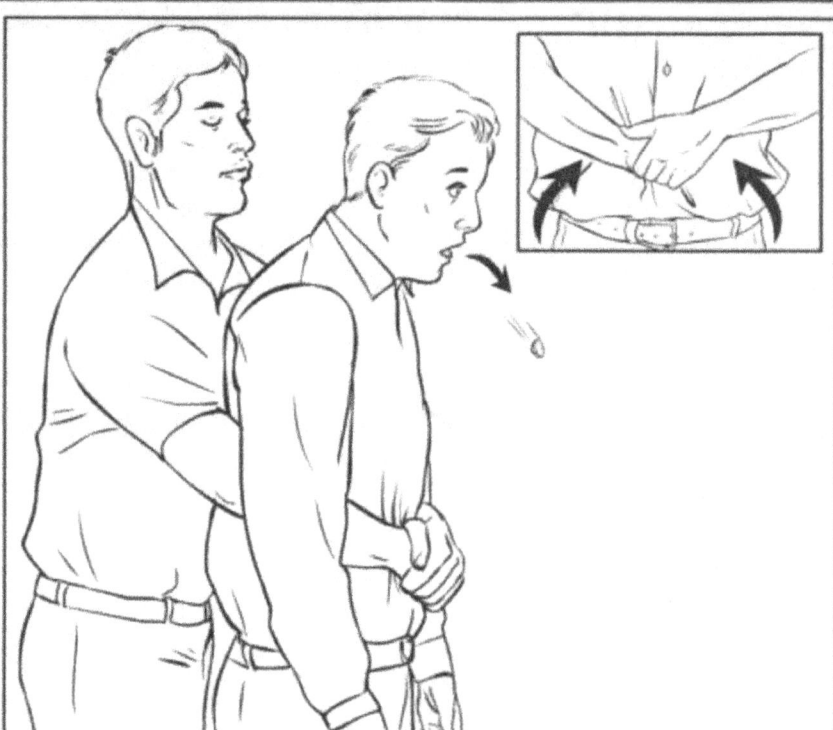

The first step of this technique is to help the person to lean forward and give him or her five firm blows between the shoulder blades. If the person is not able to cough up the obstruction, you will proceed with compressions in the abdomen at the level of the diaphragm (See Diagram on the right).

To start with abdominal thrusts, you should stand behind the person and put your arms around their waist. Five compressions are done in the space between the chest and the navel. These should be strong, firm compressions that help generate enough pressure to push the object out. While you are performing this maneuver, have someone call 911 to ensure that help is coming to evaluate the patient. Most of the time this technique is enough to unblock the airway. If the person still cannot expel the contents of the pharynx, you must wait for specialized help. Do not put your fingers inside the person's mouth to try to get the blockage out. You can push it in farther or get bitten.

What Can I Do if I Am Alone?

If you're alone and feel like you're choking on something, you can execute a self-administered maneuver. You need to stand in front of a table edge, chair, or railing and lean over.

Quickly thrust your upper abdomen against the edge. It is important to contact 911 so that they can check the airway because it may have been traumatized or fissured by the blockage.

The Heimlich maneuver can be performed on children and infants as well. In the case of children, the technique is identical to that of adults.

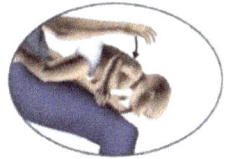
Back Blows

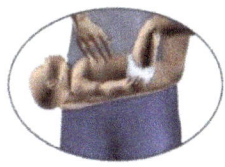
Chest Thrusts

Babies, on the other hand, must be placed on your legs face down and hit firmly on the back. You can also do chest compressions with the baby on his back.

Anti-choking devices work by creating a vacuum inside the mouth and pharynx to attract the object that is causing the blockage. They are easy to use and do not require any special training.

BruceBlaus, Own work, CC BY-SA 4.0

Tracheotomy: A Life-Saving Procedure When Help Is Not Available

If despite the maneuvers performed the person is unable to breathe, continue to communicate with the emergency line who can guide you through the process of performing a tracheostomy. A tracheostomy seeks to connect the trachea, which is the main airway, to the outside through a tube that comes out of the neck. This way the patient can ventilate if the obstruction is above this point. This procedure can be lifesaving in case of severe, life-threatening allergic processes due to inflammation of the throat structures.

a) Materials Needed:

- Isopropyl alcohol
- Gloves, preferably sterile
- Wide straw/plastic tube of about 4inches

b) Technique:

Step 1

Lay the patient down and place a rolled-up towel between his shoulder blades or under the back of his neck to extend his neck.

Step 2

Locate the soft area half an inch above the center of the sternum. At that point, clean with alcohol and make a half-inch incision. Do not extend to the sides because there are two large veins that can bleed a lot and dirty your field of vision.

Step 3

Underneath the skin, you will see the yellow tissue, which is the fat, and going a little bit lower, you will see a whitish, shiny membrane, which is the cricothyroid membrane.

This membrane is the way to the trachea; when you open it, you will be able to ventilate.

You have to have the tube you're going to use at hand and ready to use. It can be a thick straw or the frame of a pen that is open on both sides, without the ink inside.

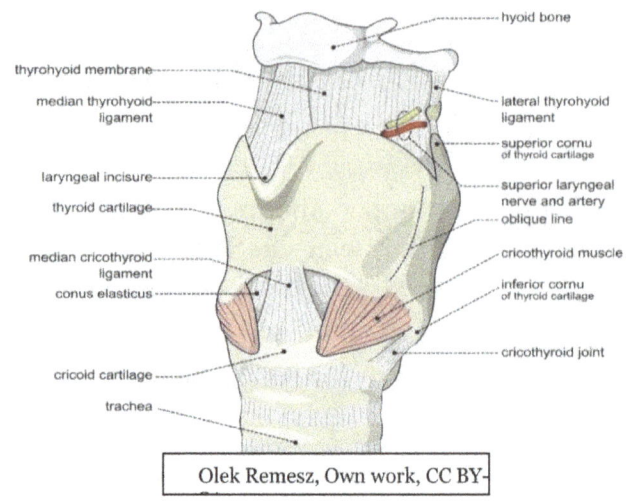

Step 4

Open the membrane horizontally by half an inch and immediately insert the tube to be used. About two inches deep is sufficient.

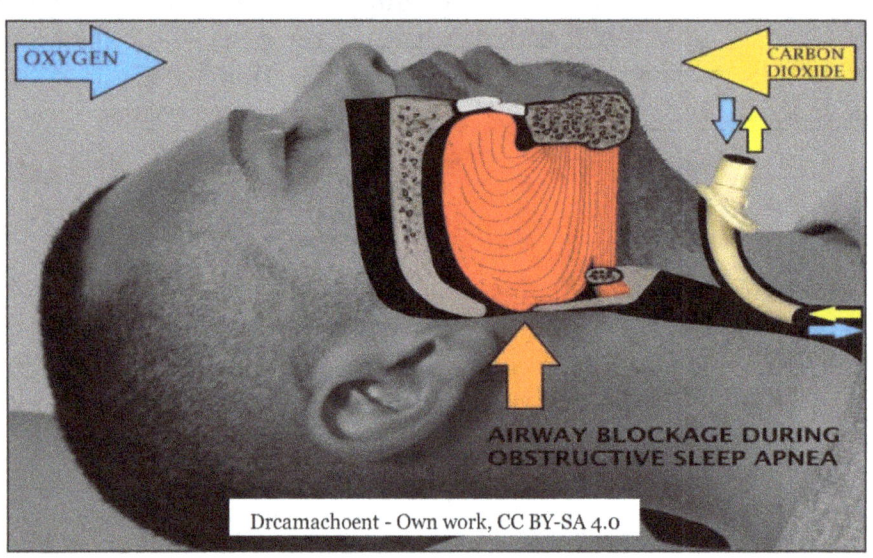

Step 5

You will know the procedure is working because the patient will be able to breathe through the tube. If there is no breathing movement, you can blow through the tube to start ventilating, as in mouth-to-mouth, but this time you will ventilate through the tube that goes directly into the trachea.

Inform the emergency line of the whole procedure and also of any eventualities so that you are prepared.

THIS PROCEDURE IS RESERVED EXCLUSIVELY FOR CASES OF LIFE OR DEATH. BEFORE A TRACHEOTOMY, MAKE SURE YOU HAVE USED ALL POSSIBLE MANEUVERS TO UNBLOCK THE AIRWAY.

GASTROINTESTINAL SYSTEM

1. Mouth Problems

The mouth is the first portion of the digestive system and is also a very important anatomical area for communication. Both the oral mucosa and the outer skin can present common conditions that are easily resolved. Dental emergencies are more complicated and sometimes require specialized dentist care.

Cold Sores

Also called "fever blisters," they are small lesions around the mouth caused by a virus. They are very contagious. Colds and fevers can be triggers, but the patient must have had a Herpes simplex infection to develop them.

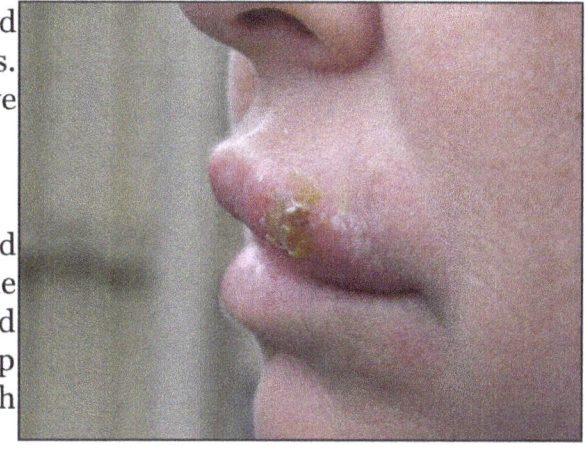

Treatment

The treatment of cold sores is to improve pain and inflammation as they are self-limited lesions. For the inflammation, it is recommended to use ice or cold compresses on the fever blister. Aloe vera balms will help moisturize the skin on the lips. Some OTC medicines, such as Ibuprofen, also help improve symptoms. Antiviral creams, such as those containing Docosanol (Abreva) or Lysine (Lysine+, L-Lysine), may speed up the healing process.

Thrush

Oropharyngeal candidiasis, or thrush, is an infection caused by the growth of the fungus *Candida albicans* on the inside of the mouth. It can commonly be seen on the tongue as white patches that, when cleaned, leave a red, swollen surface. But it can appear anywhere on the oral mucosa.

Some of the causes that trigger the infection are the prolonged use of antibiotics, poorly fitting dentures, the use of inhaled corticosteroids, and diabetes.

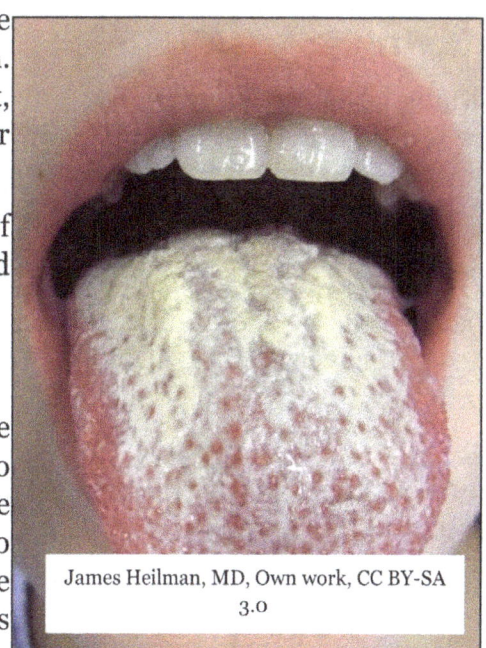

James Heilman, MD, Own work, CC BY-SA 3.0

Treatment

When the infection is not widespread, some home remedies can be used to control the fungal contamination. If you are susceptible to oral thrush, **natural sugar-free yogurt** can help control the growth of Candida in your mouth. Probiotic supplements can also do that if you don't like yogurt. If the infection is already in the mucosa, **baking soda** works because of its antiseptic properties and the change in salivary pH.

It is used as a mouthwash solution by dissolving ½ tablespoon of baking soda in 1 cup of warm water. You should rinse your mouth with this preparation at least three times a day.

Many babies suffer from this pathology. Babies' mouths usually maintain an environment that benefits fungal growth, especially when it is not customary to clean their tongues after feeding. It's hard for a child who eats only milk not to have this type of infection. A cotton ball soaked in water with baking soda can be used to clean their tongues, and in about three days, the fungus will be gone.

If dentures are used, washing them with bicarbonate will also control the growth of the fungus. Dentures can be washed with **natural apple cider vinegar**, which controls the growth of yeast. A mouthwash can be made by mixing one tablespoon of apple cider vinegar with one cup of water. However, it can produce a burning sensation in some people.

It is important to remember that maintaining a strong immune system helps prevent overgrowth of fungi and bacteria. Therefore, vitamin supplements and a diet that includes foods that meet the daily requirements are essential.

Canker Sores

Canker sores are painful and annoying ulcers that make it difficult to eat, speak, or do any activity using the mouth. Treatments such as corticosteroids and chemotherapy increase the likelihood of these sores. However, we can all suffer from them.

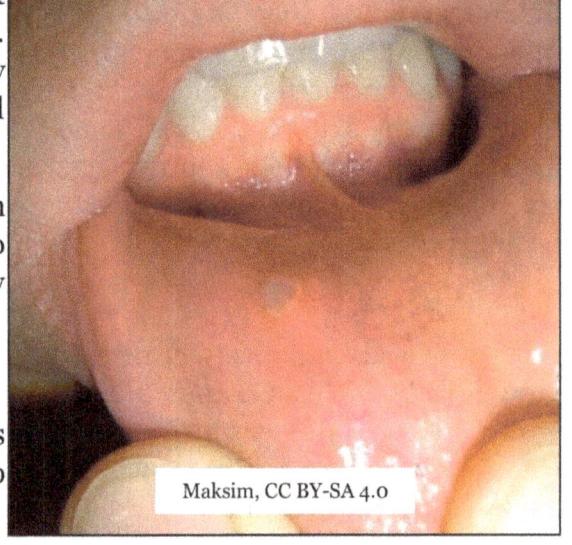

Maksim, CC BY-SA 4.0

I've always suffered from this kind of mouth injury. Although there is no scientific data, I believe that there are people who are more susceptible to developing them than others. My grandfather also presented them quite frequently.

Treatment

Although there is no specific treatment because canker sores are self-limiting, there are many things we can do at home to improve pain and speed healing.

Baking soda has antiseptic properties and alkalinizes acid that may be present in saliva. This mechanism decreases the number of bacteria that keep the canker sore open.

Just like baking soda, **milk of magnesia** and **liquid antacids** can be used as a mouthwash because they also have an alkalizing effect. You can also apply these products directly on the canker sore with a cotton swab. Remember that milk of magnesia is a laxative, so don't ingest it. Just keep it as a mouthwash.

Tea bags help deflate the area around the canker sore, improving the pain. A wet tea bag is applied directly to the lesion for approximately 15 seconds four times a day.

These methods are very effective and are not exclusive. For example, baking soda can be used with the tea bag without harming or worsening the extent of the canker sore.

Papillitis (Lie Bumps)

Lie bumps are the inflammation of the lingual papillae, and although the legend says these appear when we tell lies, the truth is that it can come at any time and be very annoying.

Papillitis does not need a specific treatment; however, mouthwash and painkillers can improve the pain. In a few days, those lie bumps will no longer be on your tongue.

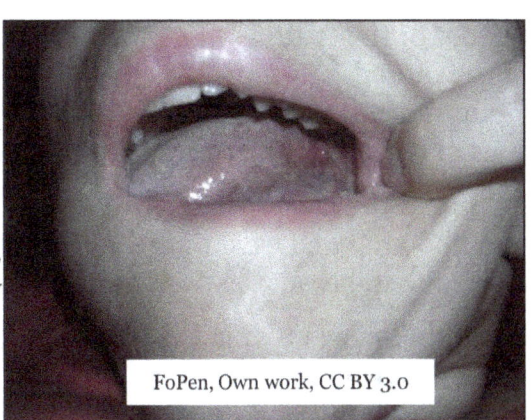

FoPen, Own work, CC BY 3.0

2. Teeth Problems

Teeth are bones connected to the jaw. They can present emergencies either from injuries due to trauma to the face, such as falls or blows with objects, or from diseases of the mouth and gums. The mouth is a completely contaminated environment; in fact, a human bite is much more dangerous in terms of infection than any animal bite.

Therefore, it is important to maintain adequate oral hygiene so that the teeth do not suffer from an increase in the number of microorganisms that end up colonizing the spaces between the teeth and near the gums, resulting in cavities.

Dental hygiene consists of flossing between each tooth space once a day, brushing your teeth after eating, and using antiseptic mouthwash once or twice a day.

However, there are situations that we cannot avoid, even if we follow all the normal hygiene rules. Trauma or bacteria that begin to grow between a crown and the root of the tooth are unexpected and should be evaluated by a dentist.

Toothache and Gingivitis

These conditions are non-specific symptoms that can be caused even by diseases of the face that are not exclusive to the mouth. Both can be very painful and annoying. The important thing in these cases is to recognize the cause so that it can be treated.

Dental hypersensitivity to cold, heat, or acids is a common cause of toothache as well as food debris stuck in your teeth and gums and dental cavities and abscesses. All these may be accompanied by gingivitis. These are diseases that go hand in hand.

In order to improve them, you must first carry out a proper cleaning of the teeth: flossing between all the spaces, brushing, and using a mouthwash. If the pain persists, one recommended technique is rinsing with warm salt water. This treatment was indicated to me by a dentist, and it worked very well.

At that time, I had a lot of hypersensitivity in two lower teeth and didn't know what it could be. To my surprise, after the dentist examined me, he told me my teeth were very clean but the problem was that I was brushing too vigorously and with a very stiff toothbrush. This poor brushing technique caused the roots of those two teeth to be exposed.

The root of the tooth is where the nerves and all the sensitive parts are, so it is protected by the gums. When exposed, it becomes very sensitive to temperature changes. The saltwater rinses helped me with that unpleasant pain that comes with hypersensitivity. On top of that, I started using special toothpaste for sensitive teeth, which I still use when I have this problem.

To prepare the rinse, you will mix half a teaspoon of salt with half a cup of warm water. This liquid should be prepared each time the rinsing is done, up to three times a day. Never keep the rinse after it has been used because as soon as it has any contact with the mouth, it becomes contaminated.

This solution is very practical and economical and really improves the problem, but if the pain persists for more than a week, you should consult a dentist.

Dental Trauma

Blunt force trauma can crack, chip, break, or knock out a tooth. When a tooth breaks but does not come out completely, the situation can wait. It is advisable to notify the dentist and follow his or her instructions, but it is not an absolute emergency.

The tooth that has suffered the impact may become loose or change color. None of these symptoms are normal, and you should consult your dentist.

However, when the tooth is knocked out, time is precious if the professional is going to save it and reinsert it. Look for the tooth, and try not to touch its root.

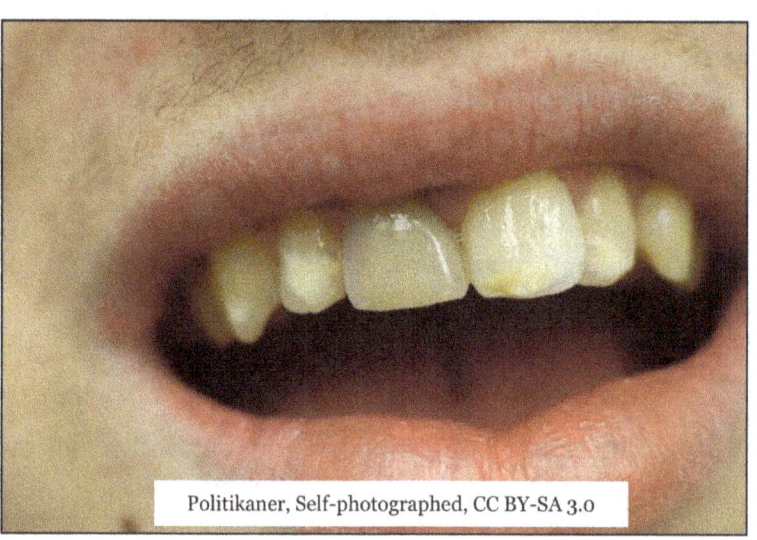
Politikaner, Self-photographed, CC BY-SA 3.0

Always remember that this is the "living" part of the tooth, so it should be kept as sterile as possible. Clean the tooth with warm water only. The best way to keep it safe is to put it back into the cavity, so if possible, reinsert it. If you cannot reinsert it, place it in a cup of milk and visit the dentist as soon as possible so that the tooth can be saved. If you can't do anything, either because you can't find the tooth or because it's impossible to visit the dentist, keep the gum clean and try not to injure it with food or your tongue. Remember that the remaining orifice is connected to the jaw. Therefore, it is important that it heals without becoming infected to avoid complications. There will always be a possibility of placing an implant later on.

Dental Abscess

A tooth abscess is a very serious problem that occurs without warning and can have serious complications if it is not treated in time.

One of the things that worried me most about the quarantine was a dental emergency. Just going out in the street was dangerous, and removing your face mask in front of the dentist at a health center seemed like a scene from a nightmare. Just the second week after the strict quarantine was declared in

Caracas, my city, my partner started experiencing pain in a tooth. The pain progressed until it became unbearable. I contacted a dentist, and **this is what we did:**

From the pain, we arrived at the presumptive diagnosis of a dental abscess. It was a pain of moderate intensity located in a specific tooth, which improved with normal anti-inflammatory drugs, although not completely.

After three days, the pain increased, and the anti-inflammatories were no longer effective. It improved only for a few hours and returned with the same intensity.

In addition to the pain was added a lot of sensitivity in the tooth, to the point of not being able to bite anything with it. Any contact, even when brushing, caused him a lot of pain.

In order to verify that it was indeed this pathology, I carried out a physical examination (even though I have never liked dentistry, but I had no choice).

With a flashlight, you must observe the entire gum to see the color and if there is a red area that looks different near the tooth that hurts. Then you should run your finger across the gum surface, looking for a lump or swelling, specifically at the site of the pain. You can do the whole procedure yourself, but it's more comfortable if someone else helps you. Once the abscess has been diagnosed, they begin antibiotic treatment and make the dreaded appointment with the dentist.

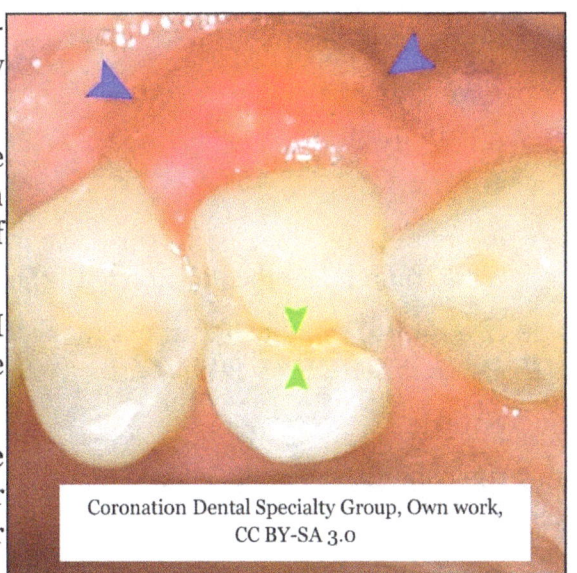

Coronation Dental Specialty Group, Own work, CC BY-SA 3.0

a) Treatment

Treatment of the tooth abscess must be timely so that the infection does not progress and the pain subsides. Although home therapies can help, there is no substitute for antibiotics. Even antibiotics, however, may not be sufficient without drainage of the abscess.

Remember that when there is an abscess, the infection is already formed. There is no prevention once the microorganism has already infected the tooth.

The antibiotic of choice is Amoxicillin 500mg taken every 8 hours for 7 days. The antibiotic will help stop the process until you can go to your dentist. Always remember that most antibiotics are metabolized through the kidneys, so it is important not to keep up with prolonged treatments, unless indicated, as this can cause irreversible damage.

b) Draining a Tooth Abscess When Visiting the Dentist is Not an Option

Draining a tooth abscess is a delicate procedure and should be done as a last resort, only if it is completely impossible to go to a specialist.

The purpose of the procedure is to eliminate pain caused by pressure and decrease infection. However, once it is drained, it is still not cured. This is only a temporary solution. The dentist has the final say in this case.

Step 1

Prepare everything you need. In this case you need gauze, a number 11 blade scalpel, iodopovidone mixed with equal parts of water or hydrogen peroxide, and lidocaine spray or cream.

Step 2

With good lighting, locate the area of the abscess where it has increased in volume and the consistencyis softer. Some whitish content may be seen. At that point only, apply some Lidocaine spray.

The patient may not be fully anesthetized; remember that the area is very swollen and the anesthesia will not work properly.

Step 3

After one minute of anesthesia, rinse the mouth with hydrogen peroxide or the iodopovidone-water mixture and then make the incision with the scalpel.

Blade 11 is sharp, so you should not make a large incision; just tap the tip to the surface of the gum. ***THIS PROCEDURE IS PAINFUL.***

Step 4

When the contents, whether pus or liquid, begin to come out, wipe with a gauze pad and press a littleto drain completely. Tooth pain relief is immediate.

Step 5

Rinse the mouth with regular mouthwash and hydrogen peroxide twice a day for two days. Visit the dentist as soon as possible.

Remember that this procedure is explained as general information because it is useful, but it is an extreme treatment to an unconventional situation.

It is not a technique that should be performed at home, unless the situation you are in is of such a magnitude that it makes a visit to the dentist impossible.

The ideal is always to start the antibiotic and have the specialist evaluate that tooth as soon as possible, even if you perform this drainage.

3. Vomiting and Diarrhea (Stomach Flu)

The combination of diarrhea, vomiting, abdominal cramps, and fever is known as viral gastroenteritis, or stomach flu. It is important to know that when we talk about diarrhea, we refer to three or more loose or watery stools a day.

Since the etiology is viral, you don't need to take any antibiotics, but rehydration is the most important aspect of the management of any patient with stomach flu.

Prevention of infectious diarrhea includes proper handwashing to prevent the spread of infection and boiling or disinfecting drinking water with purification tablets. When water is stored for a long time, even if it is potable water, it's important to make sure it's clean if it's going to be used for drinking or cooking.

Symptoms

The most common symptoms are watery diarrhea, nausea, abdominal cramps and low-grade fever. Bloody diarrhea is not common in this type of infection and usually indicates another type of gastrointestinal disorder. Also, when diarrhea becomes chronic (more than two weeks), you should think about other causes besides a viral infection.

Watery diarrhea and vomiting eventually lead to dehydration. When you have gone for a while without tolerating any food and you continue to experience vomiting and diarrhea, you may feel tired, lethargic, sleepy, and cramping in your hands and feet.

These are all symptoms of dehydration, and it is important that you begin to replace the fluid and electrolytes you have lost.

Treatment

Home remedies to improve diarrhea are varied. My mother, who is also a doctor, always makes use of this street wisdom. Her favorite anti-diarrheal therapy is to drink roasted rice water, which is a very effective treatment for improving the consistency of the feces.

Heats the rice in the bottom of the pot until it turns brown and then add water. Let it cook for five to eight minutes, and this water for the treatment. You can take this when needed. The diarrhea won't stop completely, but it will get better. However, many people, unlike my mother, prefer not to stop the diarrhea as it is seen as a mechanism of the body to expel some harmful agent. If you prefer not to take anything to stop it, you should stay hydrated.

Oral Rehydration Therapy
Rehydration therapy is the replacement of fluids and electrolytes that have been lost through diarrhea and vomiting. There are rehydration salts and also solutions that are prepared with even pleasant flavors. However, these practical solutions are not always available, and we should be aware of the recipe for homemade rehydration salts, as it is easy and useful.

In Venezuela, in order to practice as a medical professional, we have to complete a year of work in a rural area. I chose the Amazon. Vomiting and diarrhea were fairly common reasons for consultation, and we would prepare the salts of hydration ourselves by mixing six teaspoons of sugar and one-half teaspoon of salt in a liter of water.

How to Drink the Oral Rehydration Salts

Once the ingredients are mixed, you should take a sip every five minutes until the urine is light in color. Fruits such as oranges and bananas can provide potassium and may be added to the mixture when the patient tolerates the oral route. The amount would be one cup of orange juice or half a mashed banana.

The rehydration salts must be used within 24 hours. If any remains, it should be discarded. For this reason, it is advisable to prepare only one liter at a time.

If, for some reason, clean or boiled water cannot be used, it is still recommended to prepare and drink the mixture as its benefits far outweigh the risk of drinking dirty water. The recommendation in this case is to prepare it with the cleanest water possible.

UROGENITAL SYSTEM

The genitourinary apparatus is comprised of the urinary and reproductive systems. These two systems are studied as one because of their proximity and because their embryological origin is the same.

The organs that comprise the urinary system are extremely important for the maintenance of the body's water balance and blood pressure, among other functions.

On the other hand, the reproductive system maintains the body's hormonal balance that is the basis for the proper functioning of cells.

Components of the urinary system

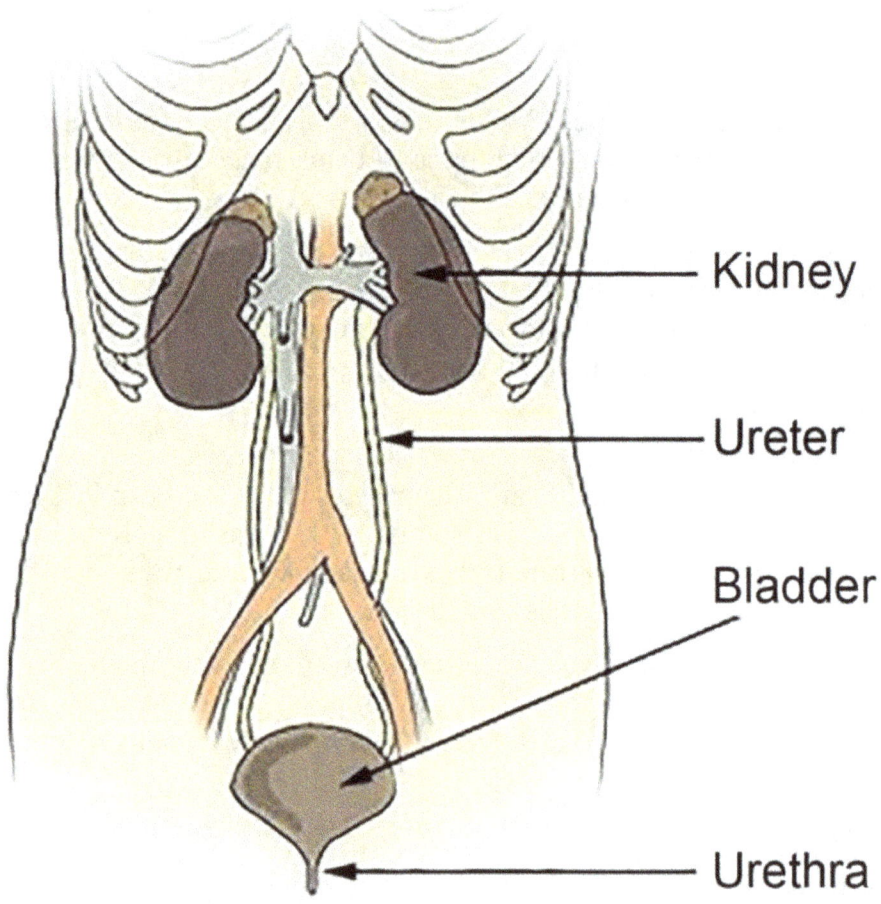

The urinary tract is divided into upper and lower. The upper tract is formed by the kidneys and ureters, and the lower by the bladder and urethra.

Female and male urethras have important anatomical differences, and these distinct characteristics affect the way microorganisms infect these regions in men and women.

1. Urinary Urgency and Urge Incontinence

Sometimes the terms "urgency" and "urge incontinence" are used as synonyms when they are not. Although both refer to involuntary urine loss, the person with urgency may hold urine until they reach the bathroom, while the person with incontinence has no control over the bladder.

If a person has either of these symptoms, we should do a medical interview and investigate the problem that is causing them.

The bladder is a muscular reservoir where urine that forms in the kidneys is stored. From the bladder, the urine passes through the urethra to be expelled from the body. This mechanism is regulated by an internal sphincter, close to the bladder, that has involuntary action and an external voluntary sphincter that is part of the urethra. We urinate and hold urine at will by keeping the external sphincter contracted.

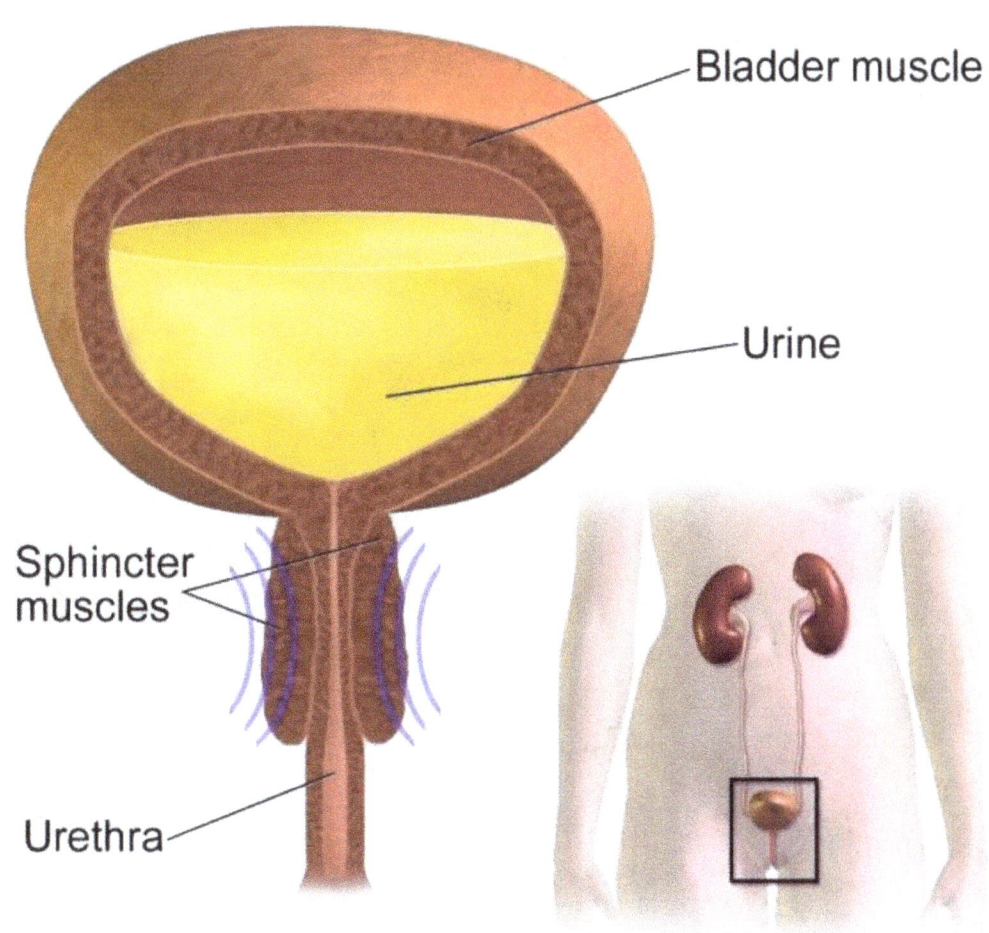

By BruceBlaus, Own work, CC BY-SA 4.0

Common Causes of Urinary Urgency and Urge Incontinence

Men and women's urinary systems are different, so while there are causes that may be common to both sexes, there are others that are gender specific.

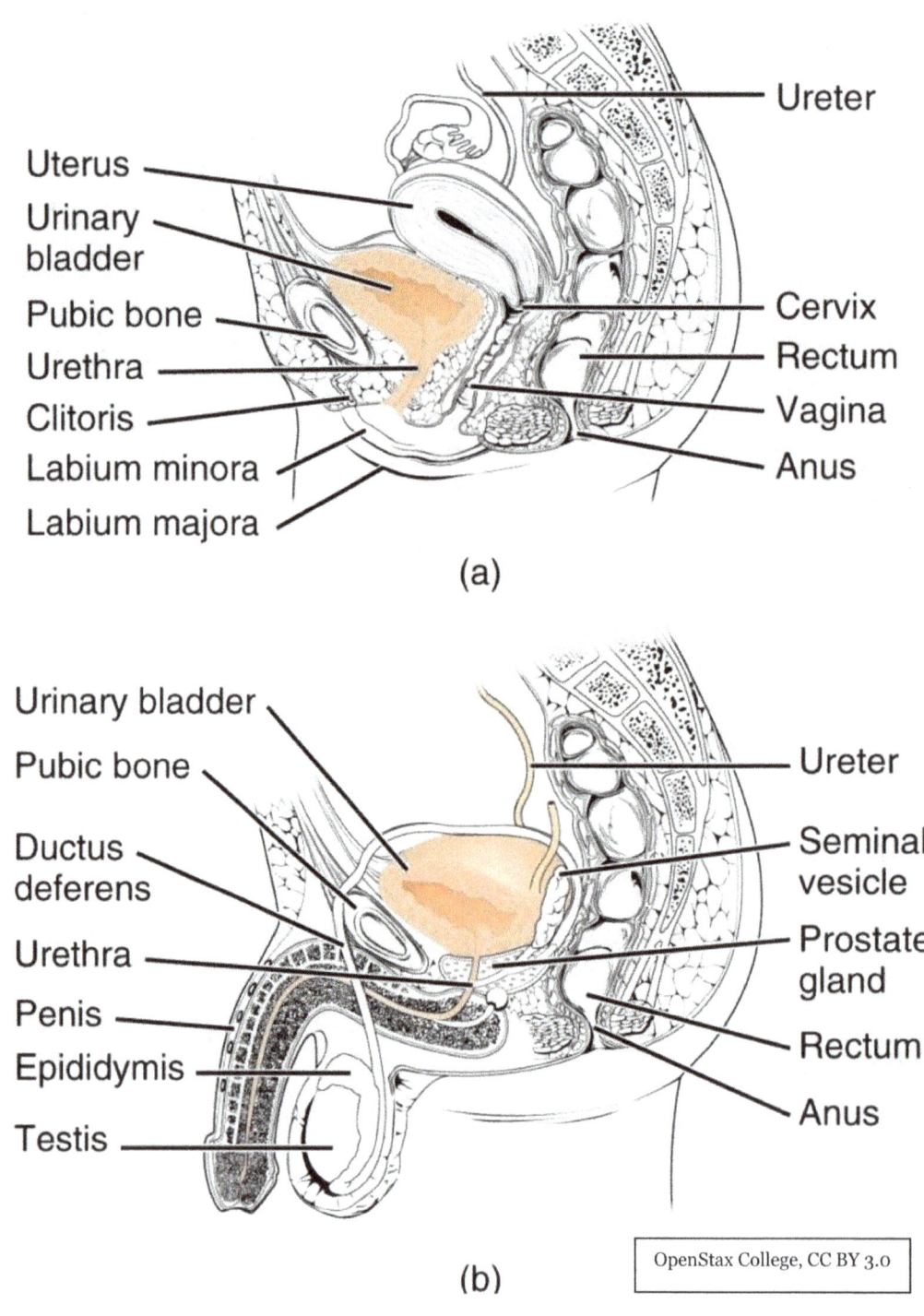

There are causes specific to the urinary system and extrinsic causes that lead to these types of symptoms. Among the extrinsic causes are urinary infections that can cause leaks because the sphincter cannot be kept closed during an uncontrollable urge to urinate; in these cases, the urgency improves with treatment.

Systemic diseases such as Parkinson's disease, dementia, spina bifida, and late-stage multiple sclerosis, as well as age, are associated with both urgency and urge incontinence. Intra-abdominal tumors that compress the bladder, pregnancy, and some drugs are other common causes.

Intrinsic causes common to both sexes are the inability of the bladder to store its full urine capacity, bladder hypermobility, and overactive bladder, although the latter condition is more associated with urinary urgency without progressing to urge incontinence.

a) Causes of Urinary Urgency and Urge Incontinence (Women)

Urge incontinence is much more common in women than in men. There are two types: stress incontinence and urgency incontinence.

Stress incontinence is associated with urine loss on physical exertion that increases intra-abdominal pressure. Stress may be moderate, such as lifting a load, or mild, such as coughing or sneezing.

Urgency incontinence is the involuntary loss of urine following an unavoidable urge to void. It represents a problem for the woman who suffers it since it diminishes her quality of life, taking into account social, romantic, and work relationships, among others.

Most urgent cases of incontinence are due to an **overactive bladder**. This condition is associated with urine loss and also with nocturia, which is an unavoidable desire to urinate at night, sometimes interrupting sleep several times a night.

In the overactive bladder, the main problem is that the pressure exerted by the urine overcomes the force of the sphincter, so the urine comes out.

There are also other pathologies that cause incontinence. One of the most common I have seen is **pelvic organ prolapse**. The bladder, rectum, uterus or small intestine protrude through the vaginal mucosa.

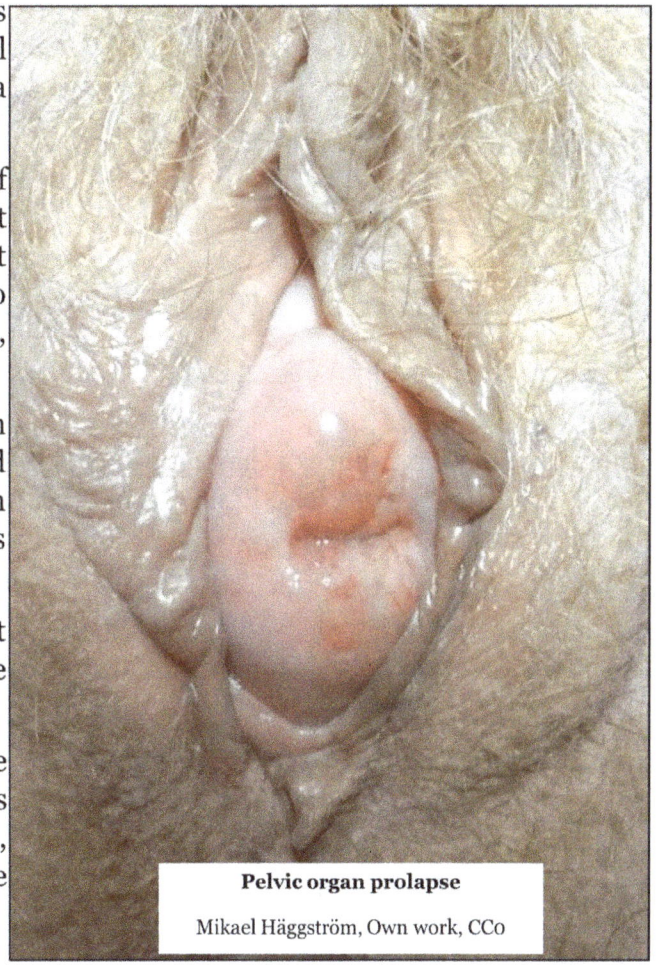

Pelvic organ prolapse
Mikael Häggström, Own work, CC0

This happens because of the weakness of the muscles of the pelvic floor that hold them in place. Increases in intra-abdominal pressure due to pregnancy, obesity, and chronic cough, among others, cause this weakness.

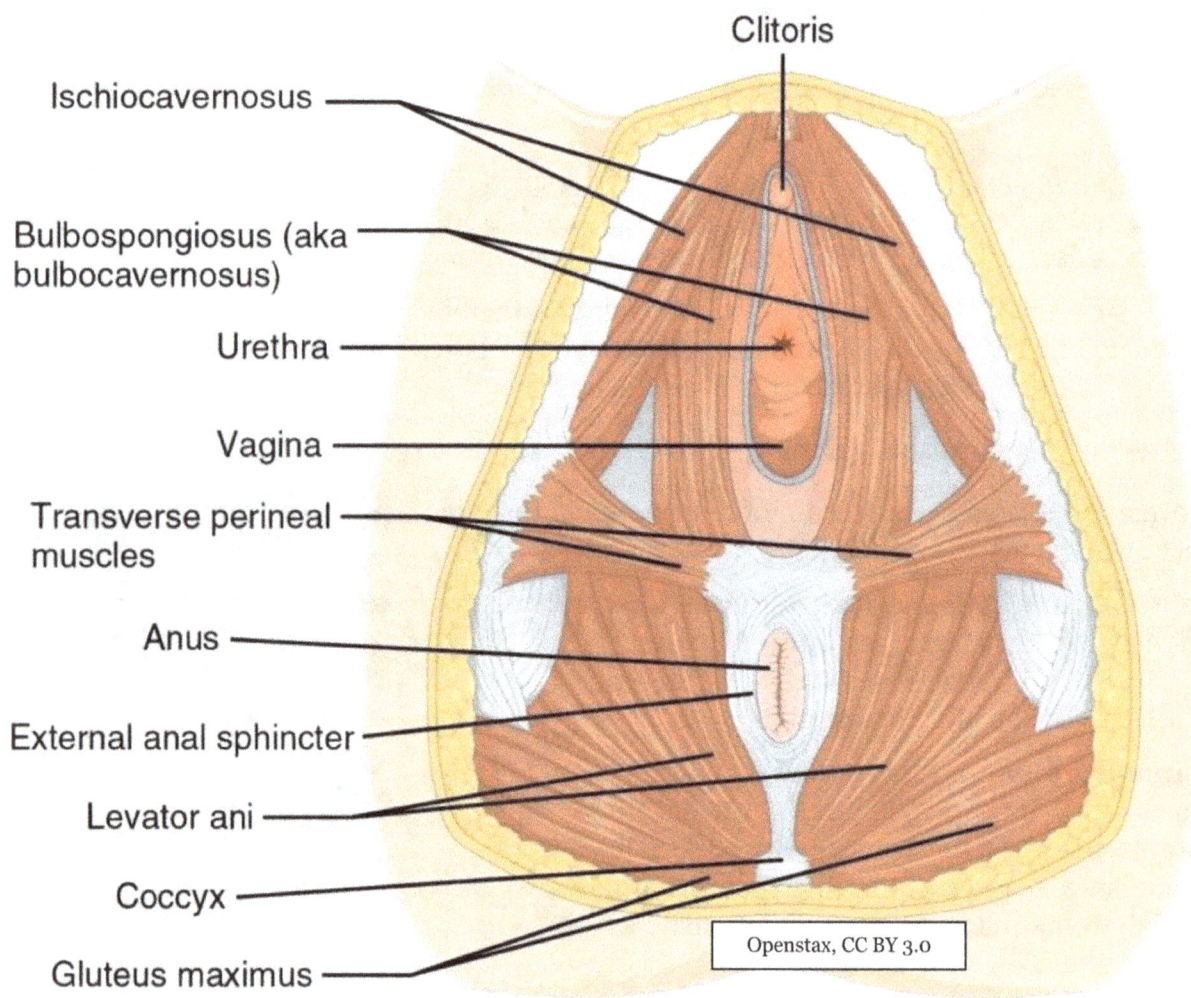

In these cases, the presence of the organ through the vagina changes the direction and angulation of the urethra, resulting in urine loss. Pessaries may reduce prolapse and are helpful for women who don't want to undergo surgery.

The curative treatment of this condition is surgical. Surgery for these cases is a short and relatively simple procedure that is very well tolerated by the patients. As I said before, urinary incontinence is one of the most common reasons for consultation in women, and organ prolapse is one of the most frequent causes.

Management

Non-surgical treatments include lifestyle changes that may be associated with the symptoms, such as drinking less water before bed or drinking less caffeine during the day. In addition to this, we must answer the patient's questions, giving them the confidence to leave behind the stigma that urinary incontinence can represent. I particularly recommend pads because they are a resource that benefits the quality of the patient's relationships.

In post-menopausal women, the application of estradiol cream helps increase blood flow in the pelvic muscles and urethral sphincter, improving incontinence.

I always recommend combining this therapy with pelvic muscle strengthening exercises. Pelvic floor strengthening exercises, or Kegel exercises, are a very beneficial treatment that helps improve the toneof the pelvic muscles and the sphincter's ability to contract and ensure resistance to pressure from the urine. Pelvic floor strengthening exercises can be performed by both women and men. In addition to helping improve incontinence symptoms, increased muscle tone improves sexual satisfaction and performance.

How do Kegel exercises work?

Kegel exercises seek to recover the strength of the pelvic floor muscles, which form the sphincters of the urethra and anus.

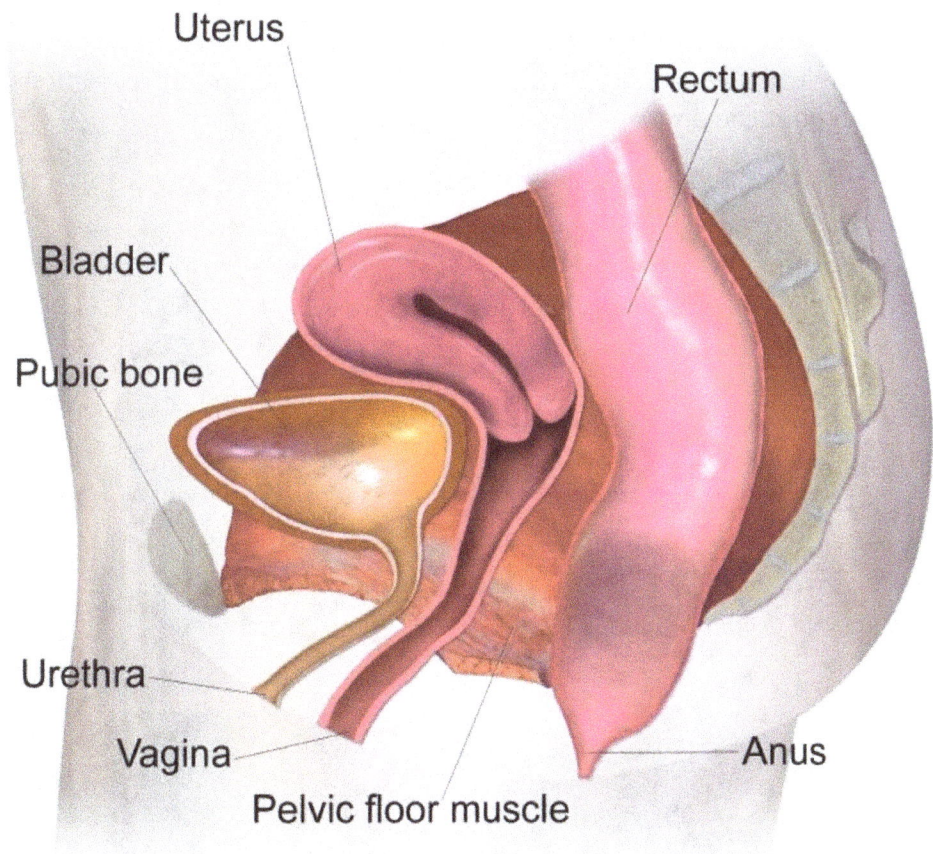

Female Pelvic Muscles

By BruceBlaus, Own work, CC BY-SA 4.0

We usually do not realize how hard we are trying to contract the sphincter to not let the urine escape. With these exercises, we try to perform this process in a conscious way so that we can control the muscles if we feel pressure or an unavoidable urge to urinate.

Although in some cases the exercises do not cure the problem completely, at least they help to control it to the point of being able to reach a bathroom without leaking.

Basic exercises you can practice at home

There are weighted objects designed specifically for doing these exercises. However, there is no scientific evidence that weight adds any additional benefit over non-weight-bearing exercise. There is no single way to perform pelvic floor strengthening exercises. The idea is to train from the inner thigh muscles to the anal sphincter, vaginal muscle, and bladder sphincter. It is important to do the exercisesin different positions so that you can contract the muscles whenever necessary without a change of position.

In the figure below, you can see three positions with which you can start training. The first one is lying down with your knees bent and your feet on the floor. You should start by slowly squeezing the inner thighs and pelvic muscles (squeezing as if not to let out gas) and slowly release by counting to ten to squeeze to the maximum point of tension and to ten to release. The second position, on hands and knees, consists of a quick squeeze and release. The last position is standing and contracting the pelvic muscles by counting to five and releasing quickly. You should try to do ten repetitions of each as many times as you'd like throughout the day.

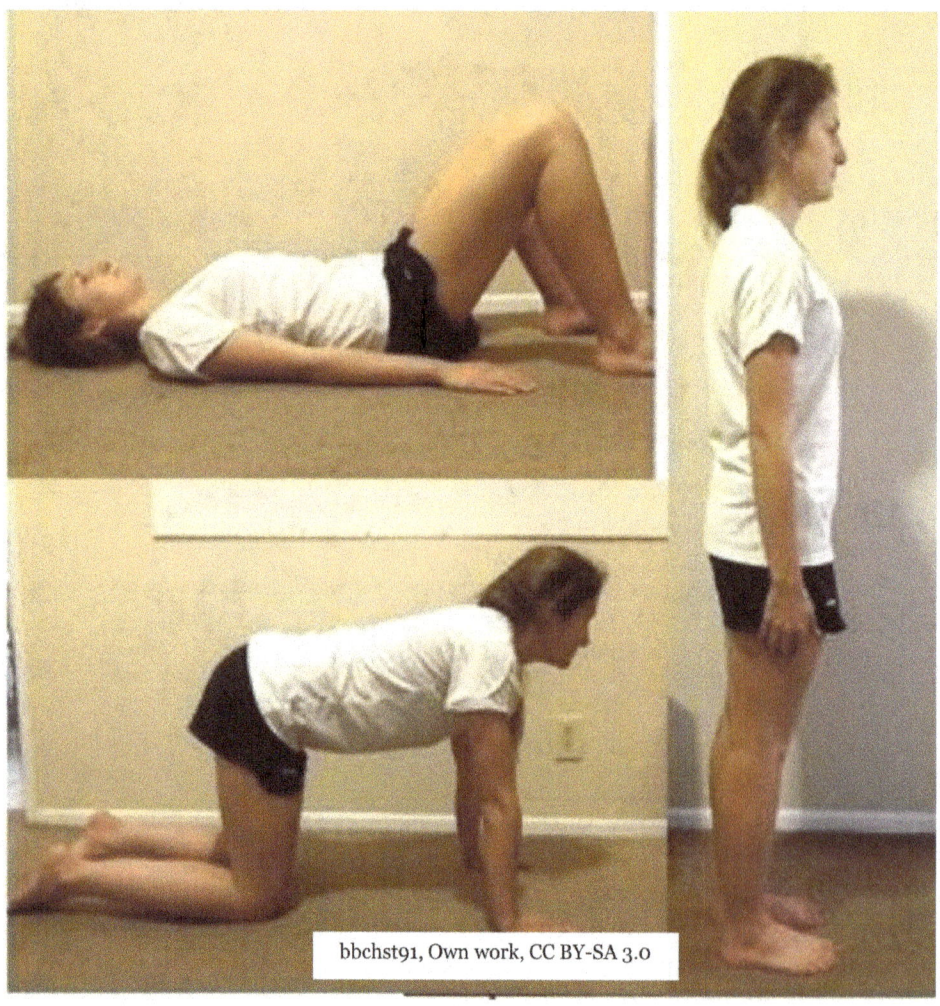

bbchst91, Own work, CC BY-SA 3.0

Other positions used are sitting and lying down completely, always contracting until the maximum point of tension is reached and holding that contraction for five seconds before releasing.

b) Causes of Urinary Urgency and Urge Incontinence (Men)

The main cause of incontinence in men is the enlargement of the prostate gland. The prostate is a gland that is part of the male internal genital system and is in intimate contact with the urethra, which passes through it.

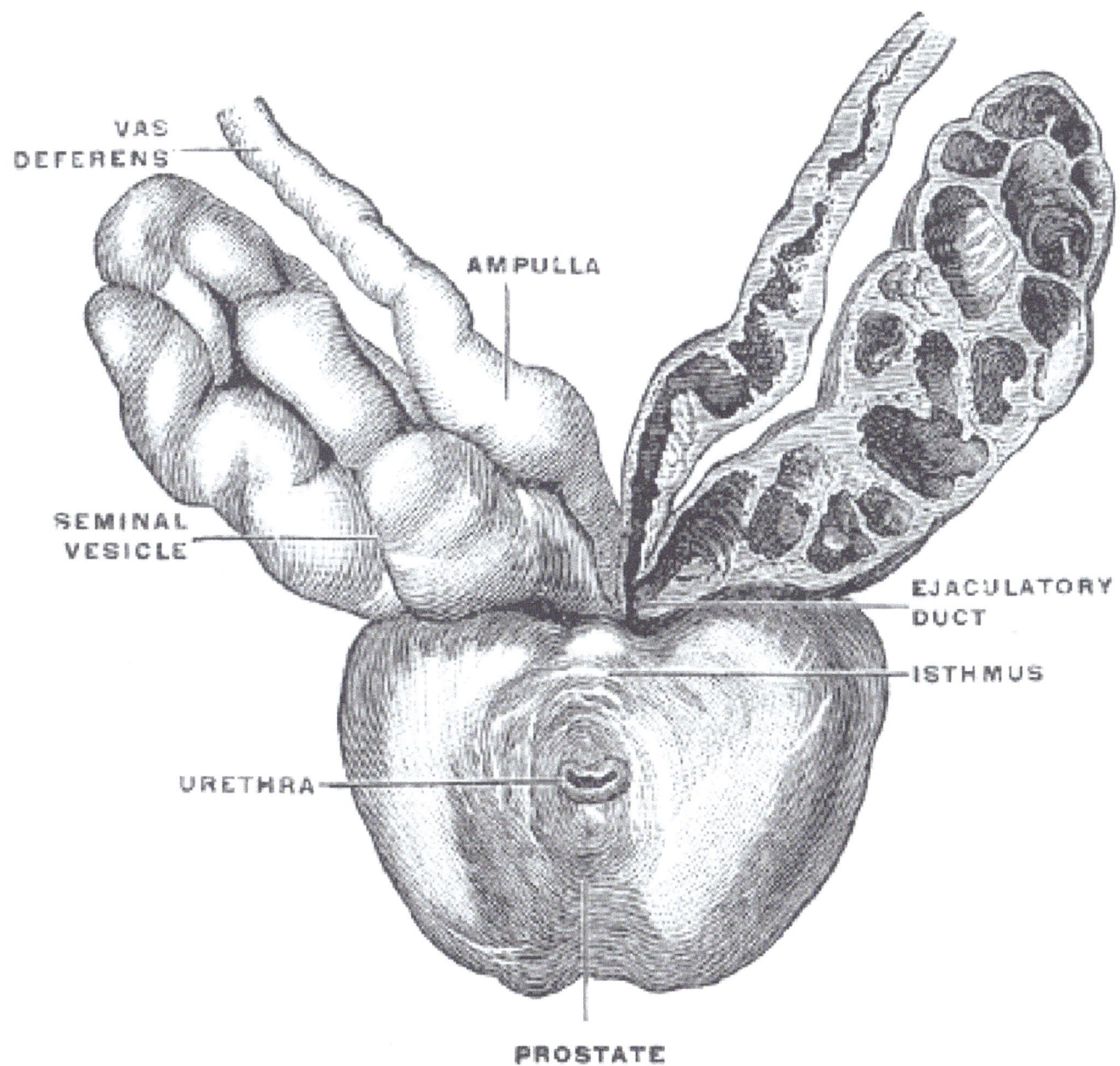

In these cases, so-called **overflow incontinence** occurs when the growth of the prostate blocks the passage of urine through the urethra until eventually the pressure exerted by the urine overcomes the sphincter and comes out involuntarily.

Other causes of incontinence and urgency in men are **stress incontinence** following some pelvic surgeries that damage a nerve that innervates the bladder and **urge incontinence** in which, as in women, there is weakness of the pelvic floor muscles. Therefore, the pressure of urine from the bladder easily overcomes the strength of the sphincter, allowing urine to leak.

An enlarged prostate is a fairly common condition in men over the age of 40. Its symptoms are mainly urinary, starting with decreased urine flow, post-void dribbling, and eventually difficulty in urinating with leakage of urine due to overflow.

Enlarged Prostate: What Do I Need to Know?

If you have had urinary symptoms like those described, it is very likely that your prostate is enlarged. The prostate is oval in shape with a central notch that divides it into two attached lobes. Its consistencyis semi-solid.

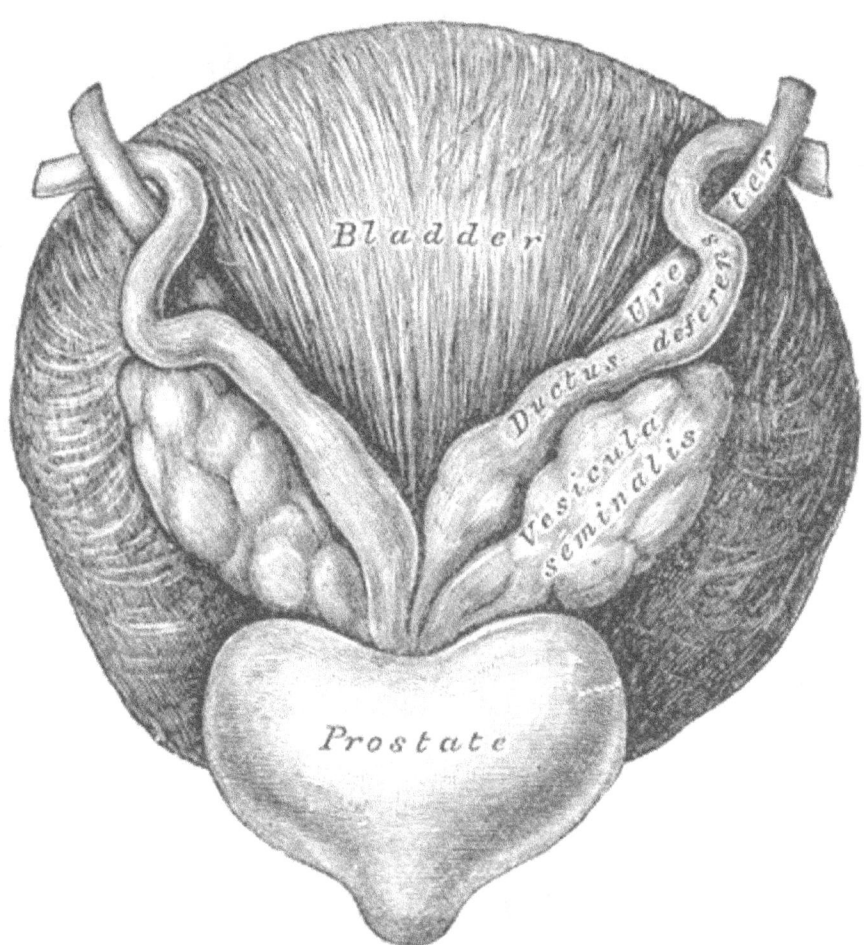

The way to evaluate it is through a rectal examination, which is a somewhat uncomfortable procedurebut also easy and quick; more importantly, it provides a clear presumptive diagnosis.

During med school, one of my favorite professors taught me the technique to rectal examination and to compare the consistencies by touching my chin, nose, and forehead.

The tip of the nose is equal to the normal consistency of the prostate, the consistence of the chin is softer than normal, and the forehead is a hard consistency, which leads us to think about cancer.

Rectal Examination:

Rectal examination consists of inserting the index finger of your dominant hand through the patient's anus to evaluate the rectal walls, anal sphincter competence, and, in men, the prostate gland.

The prostate is relatively small, about the size of a golf ball. Its consistency should be that of the tip of the nose, and its surface is smooth. You should also feel the groove that runs through it and separates it into two lobes.

You'll need disposable gloves and lubricant.

Step 1

The patient should pull down the bottom of his or her clothing, including their underwear. You can position the patient in one of two ways: standing and leaning with the trunk resting on a surface with his elbows on the table or lying in the fetal position (sideways with the knees up to the chest).

I particularly prefer the latter position as it allows the patient to relax and not strain the anal sphincter.

Step 2

With the gloves on, first spread the buttocks and observe the perianal area for any abnormalities, such as hemorrhoids or prolapse.

Step 3

Take some lubricating gel and place it in the patient's anus and on your index finger.

To lessen discomfort and make the entry of the finger more comfortable, instruct the patient to cough or bear down as in a bowel movement and then slide your finger into the anus.

The first thing you evaluate is the strength of the anal sphincter, which should be equal around the whole finger.

Then you insert your finger until you find the prostate in the anterior face of the rectum.

Run your finger over the entire surface so that you feel the groove, the lobes, and the consistency. Check for other masses in the rectum, and remove your finger.

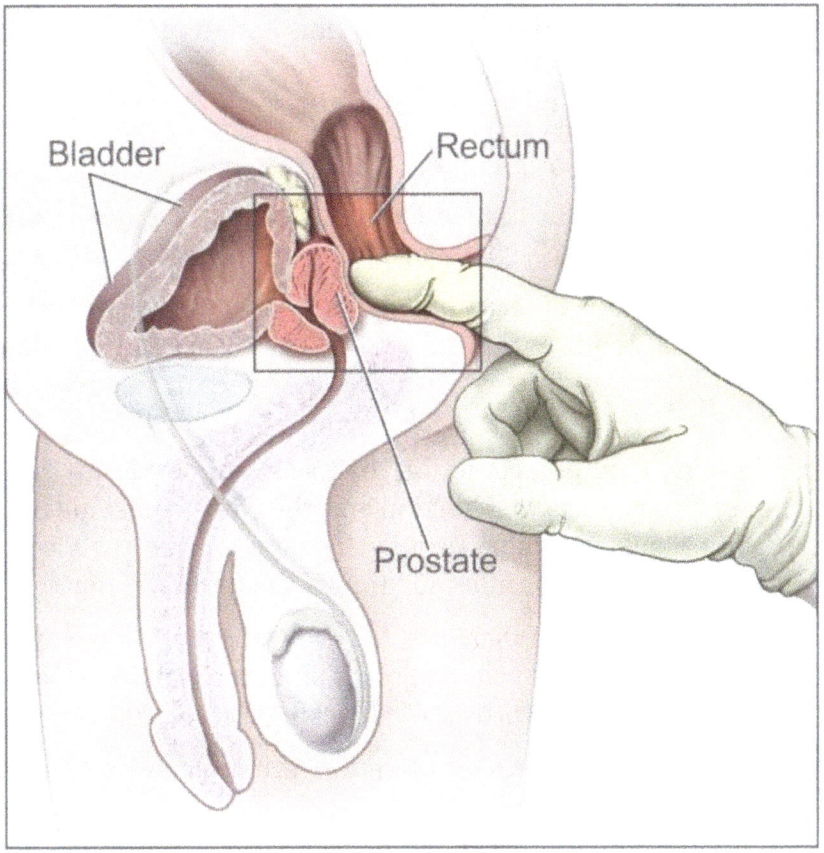

Treatment:

If the prostate is enlarged and the person is losing urine due to overflow, it is important to notify a specialist. Although there are medical treatments for prostate shrinkage, this problem usually requires surgery.

It would not be responsible on my side to recommend a medication since each case must be evaluated individually as these are drugs that have other effects. You have to be very careful with their use. However, there are natural remedies that you can use both to reduce the size of the gland and to prevent its growth:

1. *Beta-sitosterol supplements*

This component is extracted from plants and seeds to be mixed in a single supplement. Both scientific evidence and patient testimonials agree that it works to improve urinary symptoms. The dose is one capsule twice a day.

2. *Saw palmetto, zinc, pygeum africanum, multivitamin blend supplements*

All these natural extracts, as well as zinc and vitamins, have shown beneficial results in patients with urinary symptoms due to prostate enlargement. The recommended dose is one tablet twice a day.

3. *Changes in lifestyle*

Reducing caffeine and alcohol intake and setting aside time for stress reduction practices such as meditation help control urinary symptoms and improve prostate inflammation.

Straining to Urinate

Urination difficulties can have causes ranging from neurological, involving the brain's communication pathways, to local, such as bladder lithiasis. Systemic causes are usually due to diseases of other organs. Thus, there may be difficulty in urinating in the patient with a stroke.

At this point, I want to focus mainly on local causes that can cause acute urinary retention, which is an emergency that requires procedures that can be performed at home without major complications.

Acute Urinary Retention

This is a fairly common condition that, as a surgeon in my residency program, I used to see very often since one of the effects that general anesthesia has on some people is the retention of urine. Procedures such as internal hemorrhoid surgery, hysterectomy, or pelvic and rectal surgery can cause this symptom for the patient due to the manipulation of the nerves in that area.

In the case of men, specifically those over 50 years of age and those who have previously had urinary symptoms such as post-void dribbling and incomplete urination, we should think that the problem is likely that the size of the prostate is blocking the passage of urine.

In patients with acute urinary retention, a mass can be seen below the navel, which is the completely full and distended bladder.

The bladder must be emptied promptly as the urine can become contaminated and infect the patient. In addition, it can cause damage to the bladder wall and to the ureters and kidneys.

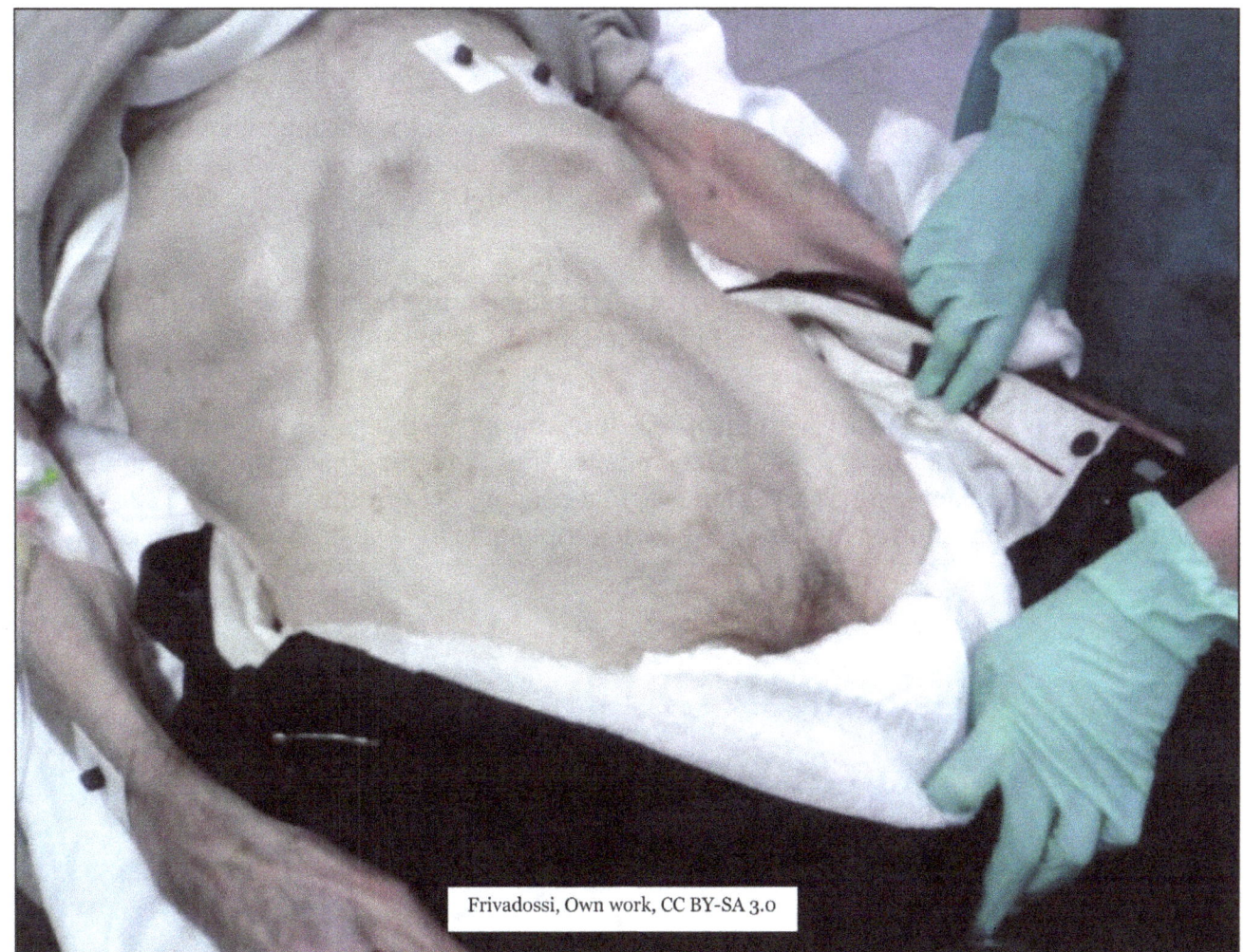
Frivadossi, Own work, CC BY-SA 3.0

Bladder Catheterization

The placement of a bladder catheter is a procedure that everyone should be aware of since it can easily solve a complex situation such as this one.

Urinary catheterization can be done to another person, and it can also be done to oneself. The important thing is to follow the directions and learn to identify the anatomical points.

Materials needed:

- Disposable gloves
- Intermittent urinary catheter #12 or #14 Fr OR 2-way Foley catheter for indwelling catheterization #12 or #14 Fr
- Lubricating jelly
- Urine bottle/bedpan/container for urine OR Urinary bag
- Povidone-iodine
- Gauze
- Mirror (for female self-catheterization)
- 10cc syringe (for indwelling catheter)

INTERMITTENT CATHETERIZATION PROCEDURE:

Step 1

Prepare all the materials so they are close at hand. If you are self-catheterizing, open three gauze pads, place a stream of iodopovidone in a container, and leave the tube half open, leaving the tip inside the package. Don't forget to put some lubricant on a gauze pad as well.

Step 2

Clean the area near the urethra (glans in men; inside the labia minora in women) with the povidone-iodine gauze, and locate the opening of the urethra. Obviously, locating the urethral opening in the penis is much easier than in the vulva.

When I didn't have much experience with this procedure, one of the things I did was to insert one gauze pad in the vagina. You do not have to put it in completely; just covering that opening is enough to find the urethral opening and not confuse it with the vaginal opening. I know this may sound silly, but it is a fairly common confusion, and you end up catheterizing the vagina instead of the bladder.

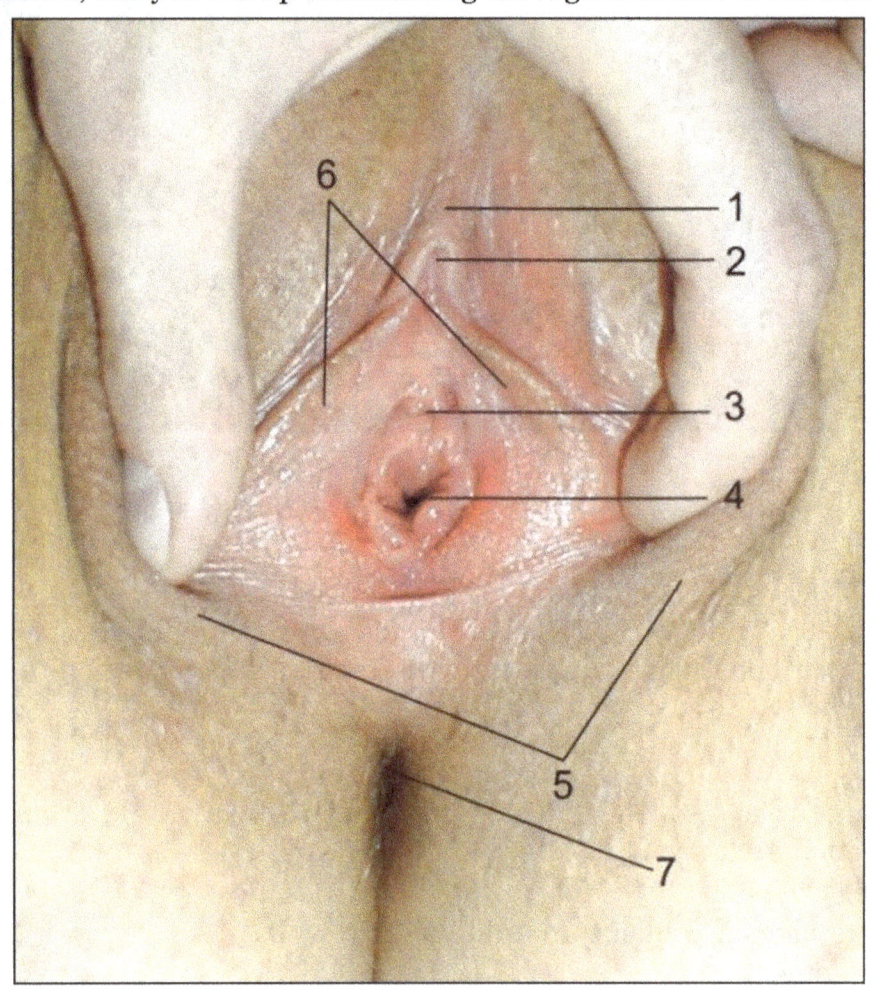

1. **PREPUCE**
2. **CLITORIS**
3. **URETHRA OPENING**
4. **VAGIN**
5. **LABIA**
6. **LABIA**

Step 3

Take some lubricant and apply it to the tip of the catheter, up to about an inch.

For catheterization just to empty the bladder, a catheter called a Nelaton catheter is used. It is made of a semi-rigid material that slides easily through the urethra.

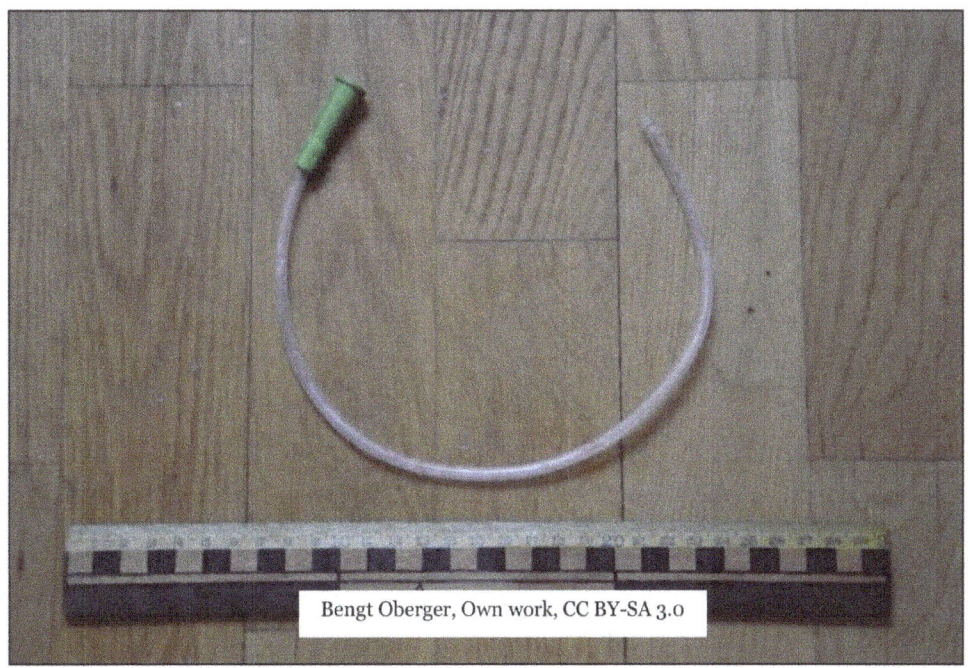
Bengt Oberger, Own work, CC BY-SA 3.0

Have the container you are using to collect the urine handy, and slowly insert the catheter into the urethra. You may feel some resistance when you are about to reach the bladder, in the internal sphincter. This is normal. Just push firmly without excessive force until it gives way.

In women, it is not necessary to insert the whole length of the catheter because the urethra is shorter than in men. To avoid spilling urine from the container, bend the catheter or clamp it with your fingers until you see urine coming out and can properly position the container.

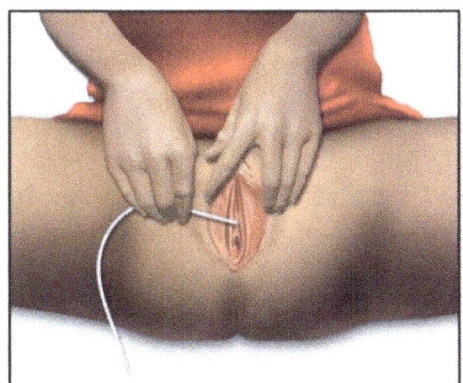
Female Self-Catheterization

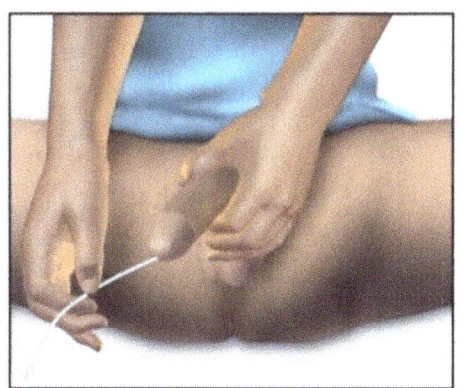
Male Self-Catheterization

BruceBlaus, Own work, CC BY-SA 4.0

INDWELLING CATHETERIZATION:

Another type of catheter is used for prolonged catheterization. The Foley catheter is the one I prefer because it is easy to use.

This type of catheter has two openings at the end that is external. One is the drainage opening, and the other one is to fill the balloon. In the end that goes inside the bladder, there is an inflatable balloon for anchoring the catheter.

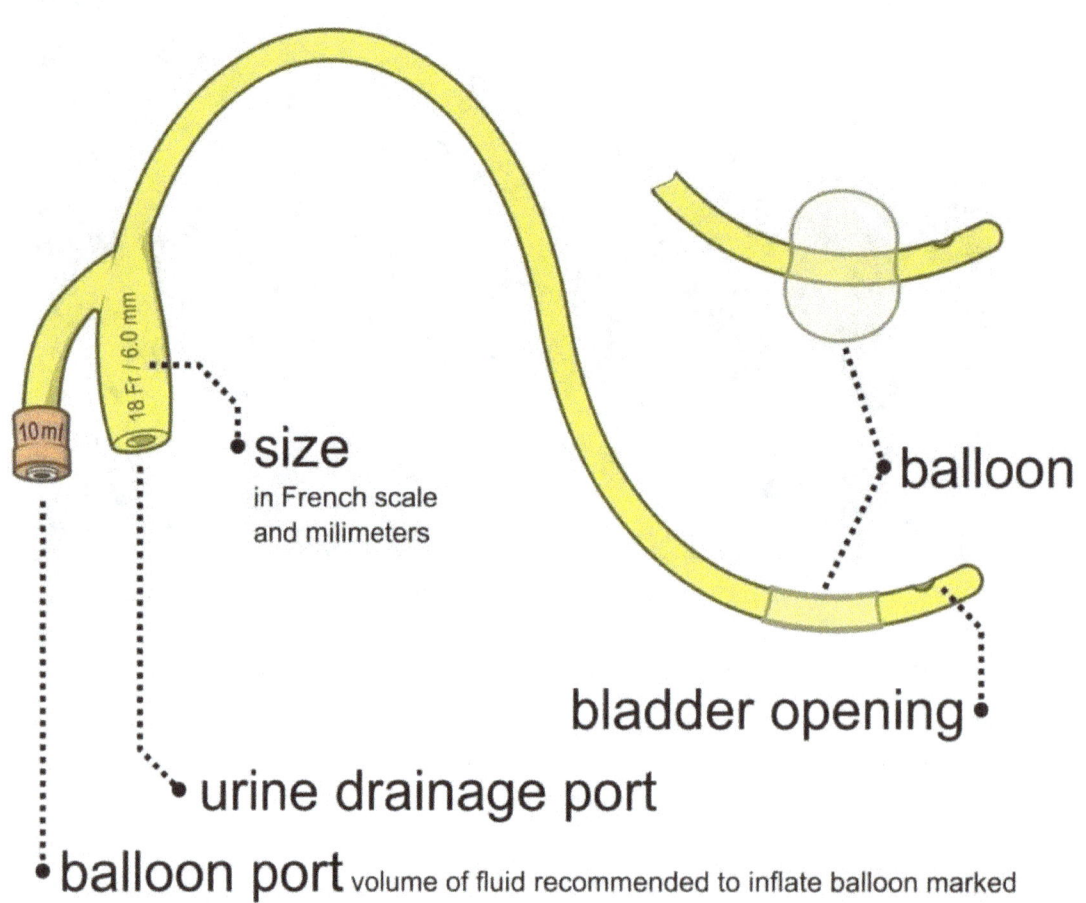

Olek Remesz, Own work, CC BY-SA 3.0

First of all, you must check that the balloon works well. Through the lumen, you introduce 5cc of sterile water or air (I prefer sterile water) to check the permeability of the catheter and the proper functioning of the balloon. Once you've checked that everything is working, you must deflate the balloon to start the catheterization.

Connect the catheter to the collection bag so that any urine that comes out falls directly into the bag. Once this is done, the catheter is inserted. As in the previous technique, in women, it is not necessary to insert the entire length. When urine starts to come out, it means that you have reached the bladder. You can then inflate the balloon.

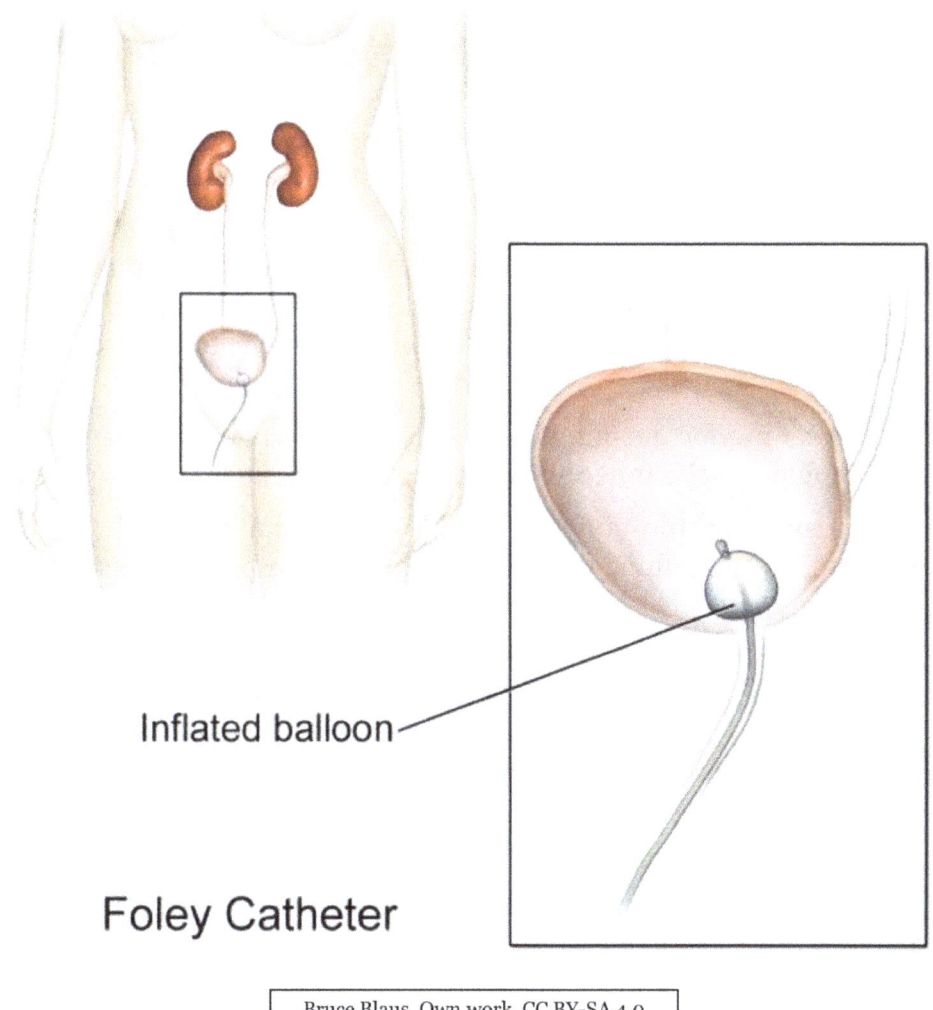

Foley Catheter

Bruce Blaus, Own work, CC BY-SA 4.0

Step 4

In the case of acute retention, try to quantify the amount of urine you emptied. This information may be important for your visit to the specialist later on. Dispose of all used materials and remember that in the case of using a Foley catheter, the collection bag should not be tightened or the drainage line bent.

WHEN SHOULD YOU PERFORM THIS PROCEDURE?

In the case of a person who feels like they need to urinate yet is unable to do so within four hours, you should drain the urine. However, always check the abdomen for a pelvic mass due to a very full bladder. If it has not been four hours but you find this sign, urinary catheterization is indicated. Try to maintain your hygiene measures to avoid urinary infections.

Pelvic surgeries can often cause acute urinary retention. I have a lot of experience with this because for a long time I worked with a team of proctologists, and this symptom was very common among our patients. Once the bladder has been emptied, the person can relax and rest. This sphincter contraction effect then disappears, and the person can urinate normally.

MUSCULOSKELETAL SYSTEM

The muscles, bones, and ligaments form the musculoskeletal system, a complicated structure that gives the body mobility, stability, and elasticity. Each bone in the body is articulated with another, forming frames that guarantee the safety of the internal organs while providing stability and balance.

The functions of **bones** are protection, stability, serving as an anchorage point for muscles and ligaments, and production of blood cells. The muscles and ligaments are responsible for locomotion and strength. Damage to any of these causes a disability in the patient to a lesser or greater degree depending on the injury.

Regular **exercise**, such as walking for 40 minutes at a medium pace or intense exercise for 20–25 minutes, is important for keeping muscles toned and active, joints lubricated, and bones in good shape.

Getting enough **sun** each day helps the body to synthesize vitamin D, which is specific to bone metabolism. I always recommend sunbathing before 10 a.m. or after 4 p.m. because at these times, the sun's rays do not hit us directly.

In addition, there are **foods** that improve and maintain the amount of calcium required by the bones and the proteins needed by the muscles and ligaments. Some of these foods are yogurt, milk, cheese, salmon, tuna, green vegetables like broccoli, and nut butter. I particularly like Greek yogurt because it provides more protein. I always mix one cup with some honey and nuts and have a super food.

In Venezuela, when you have a joint problem, whether it is pain, a sprain, or a fracture, it is recommended to eat chicken feet soup. Chicken feet have a lot of collagen and, according to popular culture, also have almost miraculous properties for improving skin and hematological levels as well as eliminating discomfort and viruses in general.

I know that in other Latin and Asian countries, the feet are prepared fried and in other forms, but in Venezuela, the favorite preparation is a soup made of this curious ingredient. Here is the recipe if you would like to try such a delicious and miraculous delicacy.

Venezuelan Chicken Feet Soup Recipe

Ingredients:
- 250 g chicken feet
- 3 carrots
- 1 large potato cut into squares
- ½ pumpkin
- 2 onionsPreparation:

- Wash the chicken feet; clean them and remove the nails.
- Cut the carrots, potato, and pumpkin into small to medium squares.
- Dice the onion, and crush the garlic.
- Soak the chicken feet in water for 5 minutes.
- Bring the water to a boil and add the garlic. Then leave to cook for 5 minutes.

- Add the chicken feet and boil for 10 more minutes.
- Add the onion, potato, pumpkin, and carrot to the water and boil for 5 minutes.
- Add the sweet pepper and salt.
- Cover the pot and let it cook until the chicken feet and vegetables are soft.

Enjoy!

CHRONIC DISEASES of the musculoskeletal system are osteoporosis, arthritis, and myalgia.

When a **TRAUMA** is received, the first protection we have is the musculoskeletal system, which provides important protection to the rest of the organs. Sprains, dislocations, and fractures are common injuries that can occur to anyone at any time, and it is important to know how to differentiate and treat these injuries until help can be sought, to avoid serious complications.

1. Osteoporosis

Osteoporosis is the progressive depletion of bone minerals that makes bones week and prone to injury.

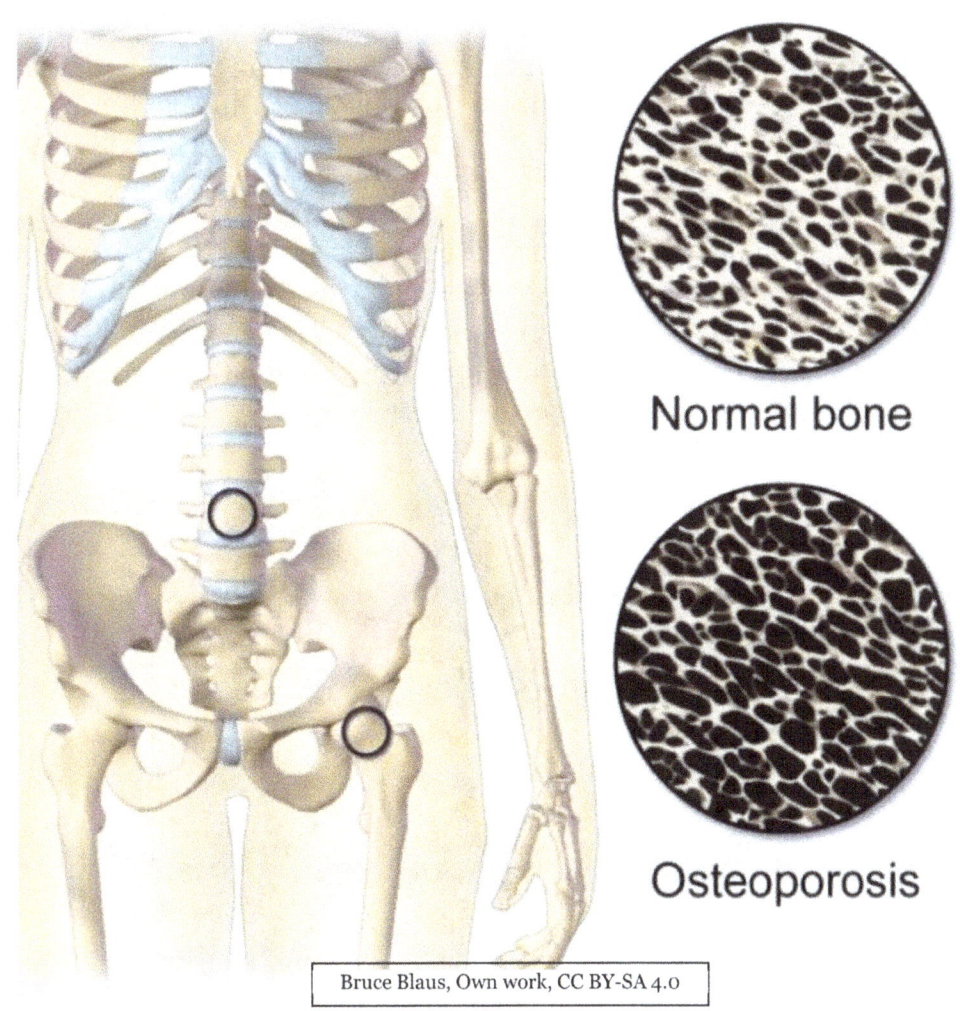

Bruce Blaus, Own work, CC BY-SA 4.0

Age and sex are two of the main triggers of this condition. Women are at much greater risk for this condition, and I recommend always taking a calcium supplement from the age of 45.

In addition, menopause and treatments that eliminate female hormones, like some chemotherapy drugs, accelerate the process of osteoporosis.

Diagnosing the disease in its early stages is difficult because it does not have pronounced symptoms. There may be pain in the limbs and joints and some weakness. In the bone density test, we can objectively see the percentage of mineral in the bones and their risk of osteoporosis and fracture.

Preventive therapy is always the best option to avoid developing osteoporosis. However, if it has not been possible or your demineralization has advanced rapidly because of menopause, bariatric surgery, or some medication, there are treatments that can help.

Treatments other than calcium supplements are by prescription and are called bisphosphonates; these include Alendronate (Binosto, Fosamax), Risedronate (Actonel, Atelvia), Ibandronate (Boniva), and Zoledronic acid (Reclast, Zometa).

2. Arthritis

Arthritis encompasses a group of progressive diseases characterized by pain and inflammation of the joints. The most common types are rheumatoid arthritis, osteoarthritis, and gout.

Rheumatoid Arthritis

Rheumatoid arthritis is an autoimmune, hereditary disease that affects the body's joints but also has clinical manifestations in other organs, such as the skin and eyes. In addition to pain and decreased mobility and elasticity, arthritis causes deformity of the joints.

It is very common to see elderly people with deformity of the fingers that have thickened knuckles; these signs are typical of the disease.

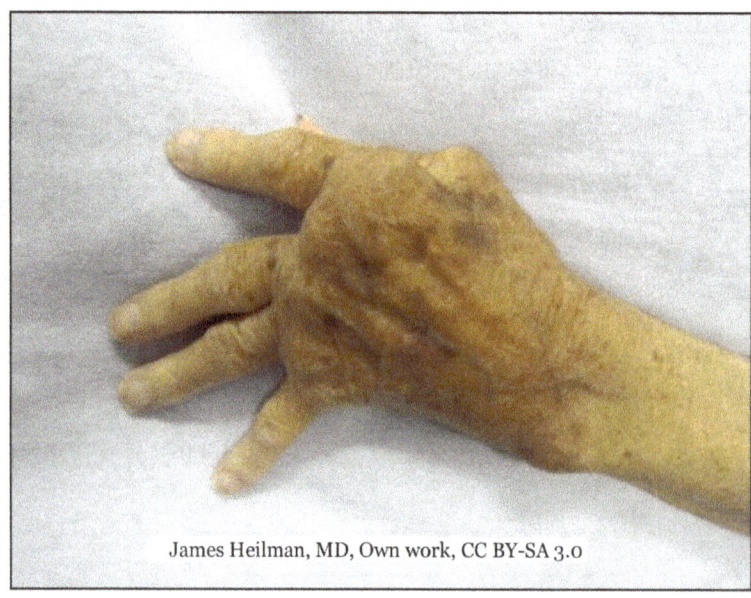
James Heilman, MD, Own work, CC BY-SA 3.0

There is a subtype called "juvenile" rheumatoid arthritis that occurs in children and adolescents up to age 16. The diagnosis is made from the patient's clinic and is corroborated with x-ray images and specific blood tests to find the genetic variation.

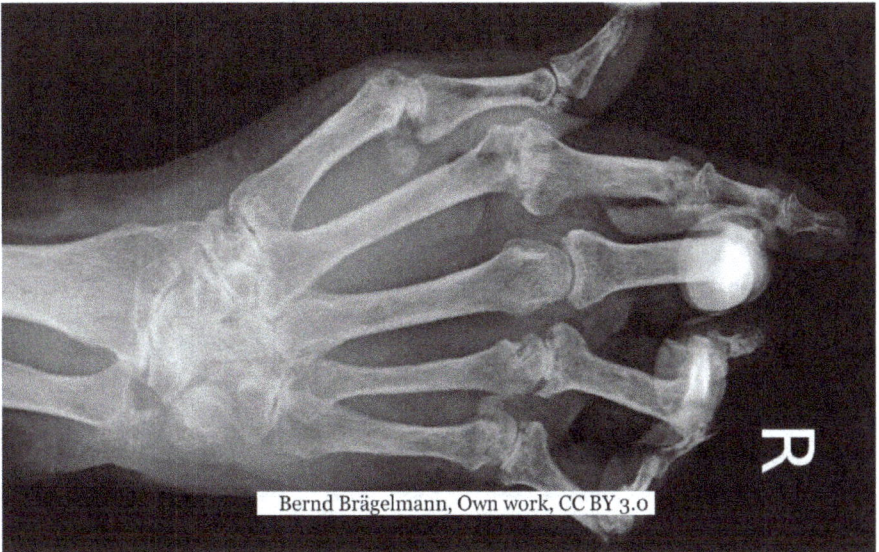
Bernd Brägelmann, Own work, CC BY 3.0

There is no prevention or cure for rheumatoid arthritis. Treatments to manage it are quite effective and slow the progression. Hydroxychloroquine is one of the most widely used medications. It is an antimalarial that has anti-inflammatory and immunological properties. This treatment should be strictly followed by your doctor as it has cardiovascular side effects.

DO NOT USE HYDROXYCHLOROQUINE WITHOUT MEDICAL SUPERVISION.

Nonsteroidal anti-inflammatory drugs (NSAIDs) are used for pain crises along with topical creams that can help inflammation. I do not recommend my patients use NSAIDs on a prolonged basis because of their gastric repercussions. I prefer to recommend natural therapies, such as rosemary, honey, ginger, and turmeric. Whether as an infusion or in capsules as a dietary supplement, these products are powerful anti-inflammatories.

Osteoarthritis

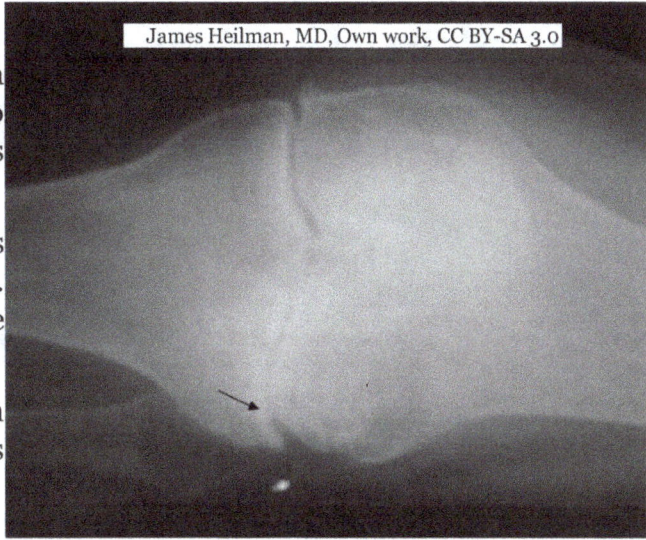
James Heilman, MD, Own work, CC BY-SA 3.0

Osteoarthritis, also known as arthrosis, is a progressive degenerative disease that occurs due to the wearing away of the bony and cartilaginous structures of the joints.

Despite its similarity to arthritis, it does not share its genetic etiology or extra-articular manifestations. Osteoarthritis is limited to the joints, especially those that support weight, such as the knees and ankles.

The main cause is age, but osteoarthritis is also seen in high-performance athletes who overload the joints and in dancers, the latter presenting it in the hip. In addition to symptoms such as progressive pain in a specific joint and lack of elasticity and range of movement, the diagnosis is made with a simple x-ray of the painful joint and MRI.

Omega-3 supplements, salmon, avocado, and turmeric provide great benefits for the symptoms of this condition.

Omega-3 capsules: 1 daily as prevention or if you are already diagnosed

The combination of Chondroitin and Glucosamine is also therapy that presents benefits that although not scientifically proven, are certified by testimonials.

Glucosamine Chondroitin Turmeric tablets: 1 daily if you have symptoms or are diagnosed

Special cases, such as athletes or people who are disabled by joint pain or blockage, are treated with replacement surgery of the affected joint. My recommendation is always to take the supplements and to exercise to avoid or slow down the wearing process.

Gout

Gout is an inflammatory disease of the joints that is caused by the accumulation of crystals of a blood product called uric acid. Uric acid is normally found in the circulation as a product of the metabolization of some foods by the liver. When it is in higher than normal amounts, it cannot be excreted and instead crystallizes. These crystals end up in the joints, causing a lot of pain.

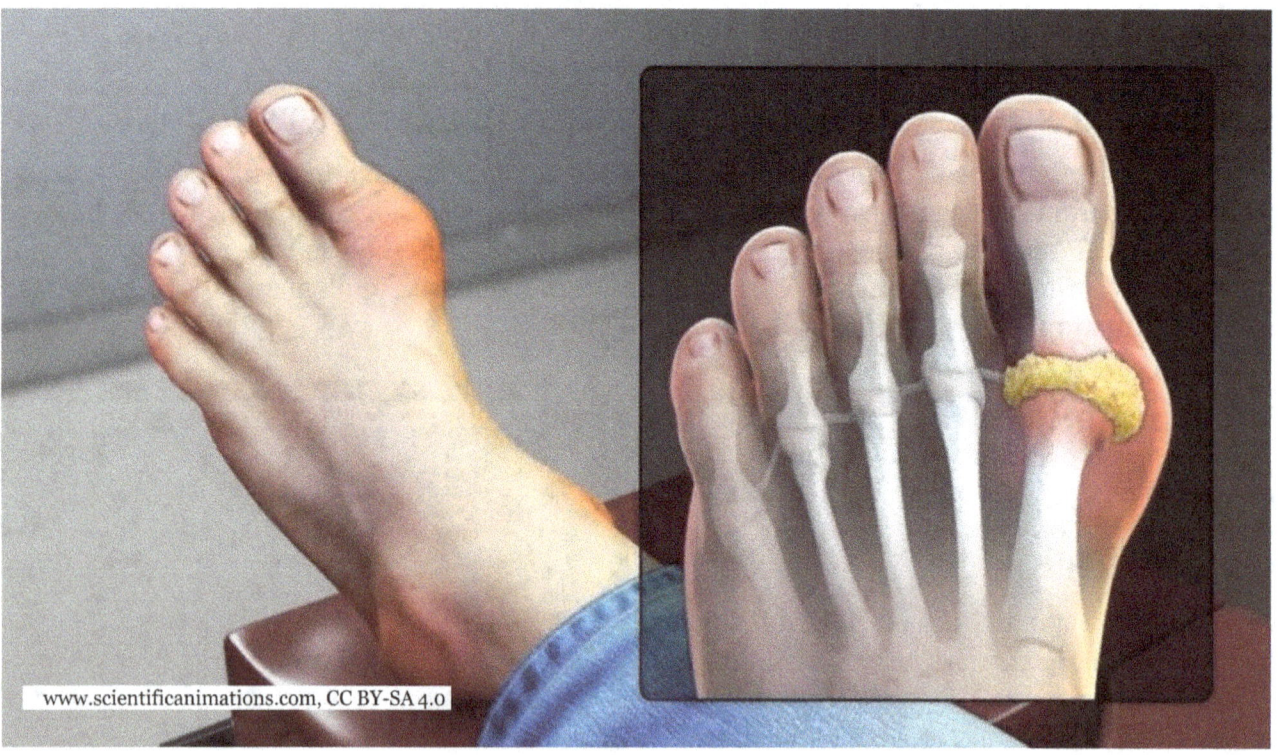

www.scientificanimations.com, CC BY-SA 4.0

Gout is known as the "rich man's disease" because its appearance is associated, among other factors, with meat consumption. The joint most often affected is the one at the base of the first toe, where you can see increased volume, redness, and increased temperature. The pain settles in less than an hour and becomes very intense. Painful episodes can last up to 24 hours.

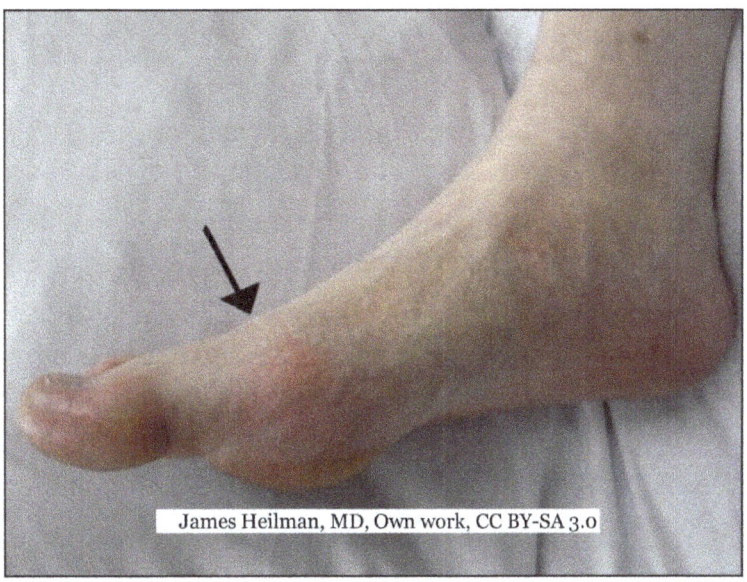

Gout may have extra-articular symptoms, such as gouty tophi on the arms and ears.

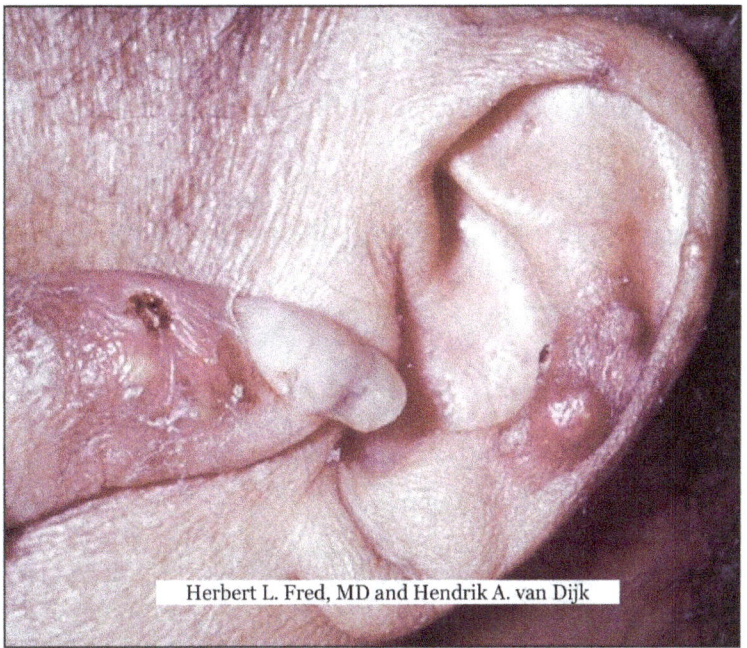

Although most patients with gout have only one attack during a year, a percentage have chronic episodes of pain that wear down the joints.

Once again, I recommend a natural anti-inflammatory. Ginger, turmeric, and honey help in this kindof process. Specifically, for gout, the cherry has been widely studied, and it is recommended.

If you don't like cherries, there are many supplement options that you can add to your normal diet.

Cherry softgels: 1 daily

3. Muscle Pain (Myalgia)

Muscle pain encompasses a range of conditions that may or may not be pathological. Strong physical activity, playing new sports, and sitting for a long time are examples of causes of muscle pain.

Viral diseases are very often associated with pain in the musculoskeletal system, especially myalgia. Infections such as the flu and the common cold can cause almost disabling muscle pain.

In Venezuela and all Latin America, dengue fever is a very frequent viral infection in which myalgia is part of the clinical picture. It is so intense that there is skin hypersensitivity. I can certify these symptoms from my own experience with two dengue infections that kept me in bed for a week each.

Muscle injury is a common cause of pain in athletes and construction workers. Having practiced CrossFit, injuries such as muscle hematoma and abscess were very common in the gym.

Whether from overuse and abuse of the muscle when trying to lift heavy loads or injuries from direct blows to the muscle from the bars and discs, on more than one occasion, these caused severe muscle hematoma to my teammates.

Muscle Hematoma

A hematoma within the muscle is an accumulation of blood that forms from the rupture or tearing of the muscle, usually from a direct blow to the muscle.

On physical examination, much swelling is evident with an intense black to violet bruise, which is very painful and disabling to the patient. Treatment includes immobilization of the limb with anti-inflammatory therapy and even corticosteroids.

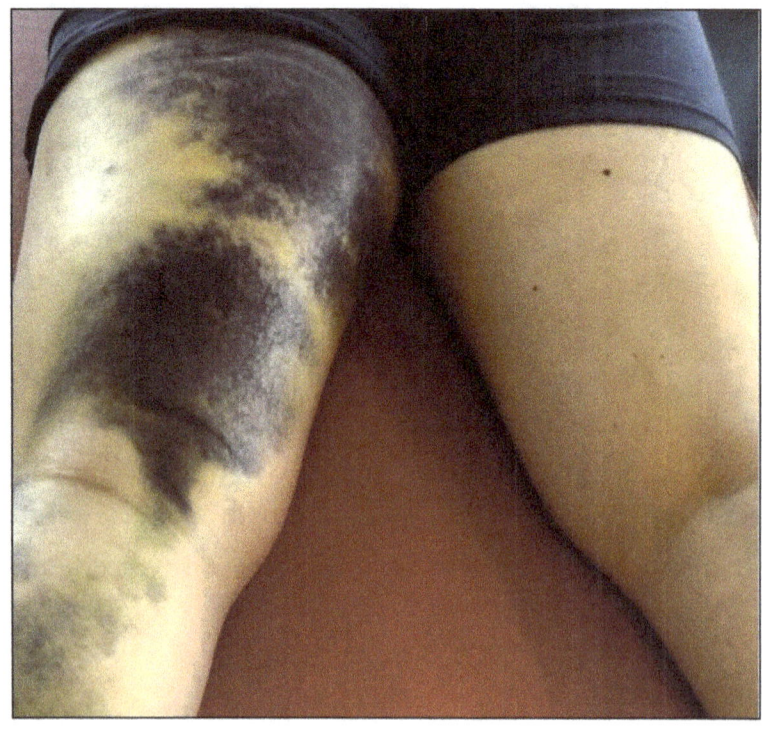

This type of injury can be complicated by a serious condition called **compartment syndrome**, in which increased pressure within the muscle causes decreased blood supply to the entire limb, threatening its vitality.

This is why it is very important to treat this type of injury in a timely manner and to assess its evolution. Further physical therapy is especially important for the athlete. Eating quality proteins, such as lean meat, or grains, such as lentils, helps regenerate muscle damage.

If you see an intramuscular hematoma like the one in the image, you should evaluate the circulation of the limb. The easiest way is to look at the capillary filling, which is how fast the blood fills the nail bed. All you have to do is press a little on the nail and release to observe how long it takes to fill up again. The filling time should take less than 2 seconds.

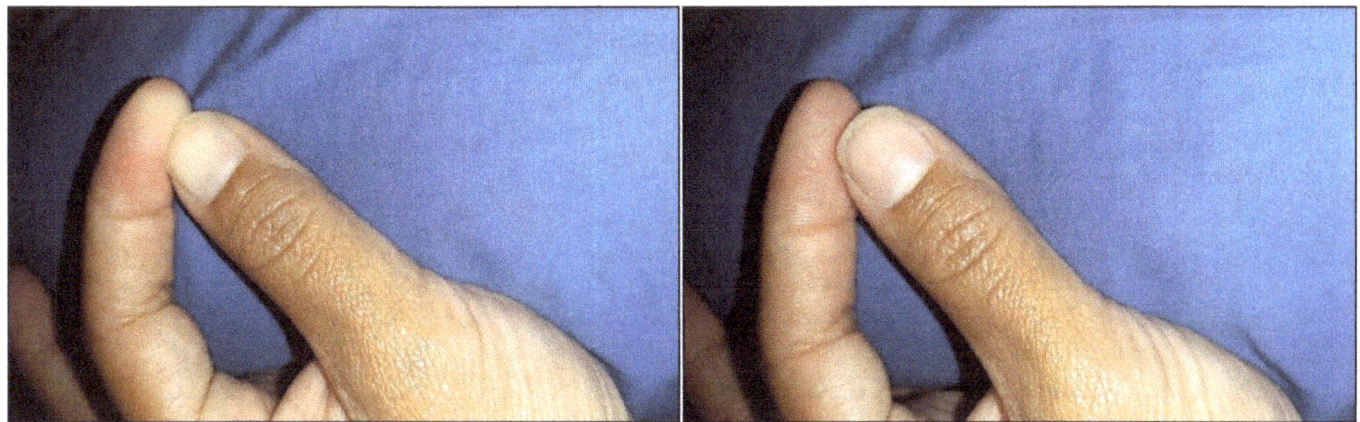

Capillary filling is the result of circulation through the entire limb. It is a simple test that provides a lotof information. If the capillary filling takes too long and the nail bed looks pale, it is important to seek help because there may be vascular involvement from the swelling in the muscle.

Muscle Abscess

Muscle abscess is another complication that can occur after an intra-muscular hematoma. However, in addition to traumatic causes, there may be muscular bruising due to infection, especially in diabetic patients, HIV positive patients, and those who, for whatever reason, have a decreased immune system.

All muscle abscesses require intravenous antibiotic therapy for at least a few days to prevent necrosis of the nearby tissues.

When I worked in Amazonas, I had the opportunity to treat several patients with this pathology, caused by snakebite. When they went out hunting at night, it was not uncommon for them to suffer minor attacks from some animals.

In these cases, depending on the symptoms, I would inject corticosteroids, and begin therapy with antibiotics for three days. I would then continue with oral Ciprofloxacin 500 mg, every 12 hours for 10 days. I never had to attend to a poisonous snake bite, but I always had antiophidic serum so I don't think it would have been a major problem.

4. Sprain

A sprain is an injury to the ligaments of a joint by their sudden and excessive stretching with torsion. It is characterized by severe pain, much swelling of the affected area, and sometimes bruising of the skin.

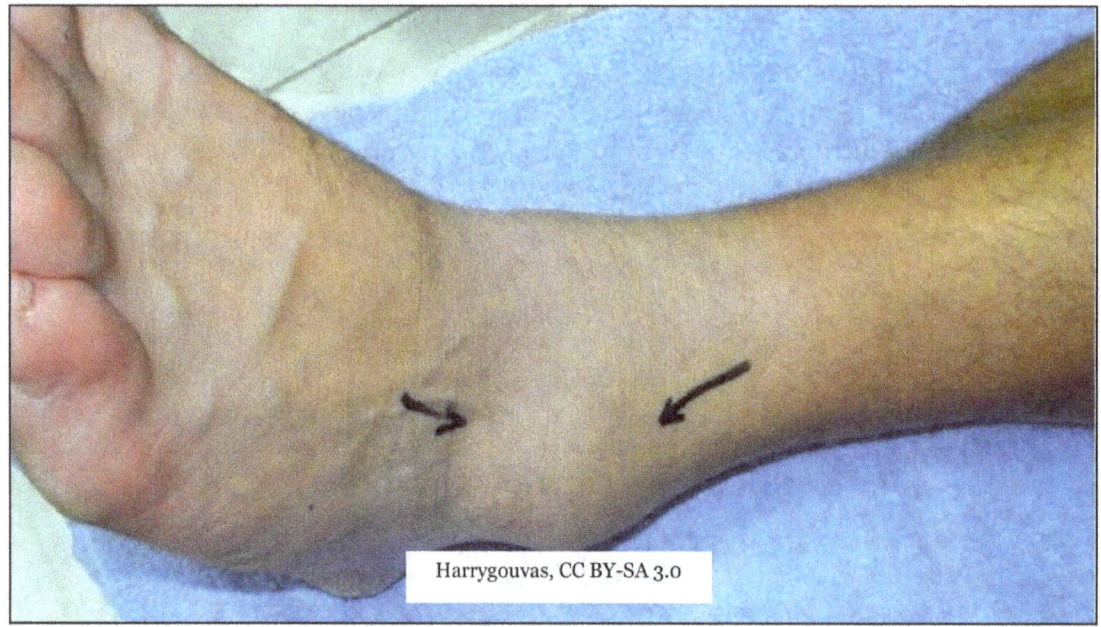
Harrygouvas, CC BY-SA 3.0

There may be a genetic predisposition to sprains, but these usually occur when there is an overload of the joints. Being among athletes, I realized that this is a very common injury that even coaches learn to handle when they are mild. There are **three degrees** of strain depending on the severity of the injury:

FIRST DEGREE SPRAIN

This is a minor stretching injury with swelling and moderate pain.

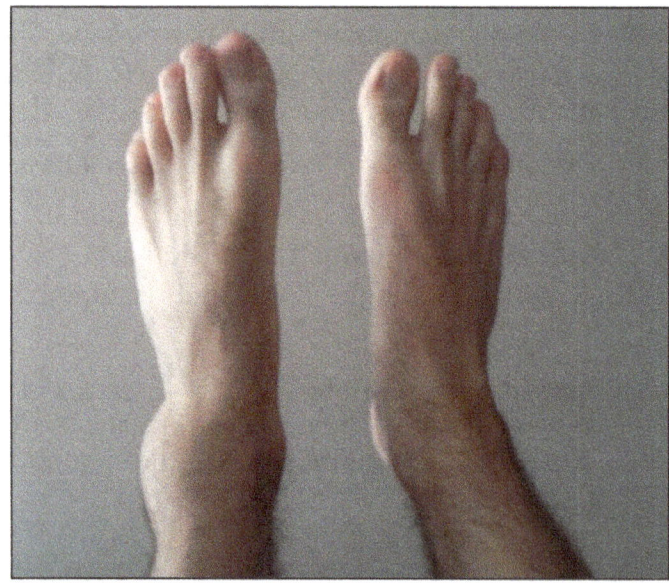

SECOND DEGREE SPRAIN

There is partial tearing of the ligament, and the patient has pain, swelling, bruising, and some instability in walking.

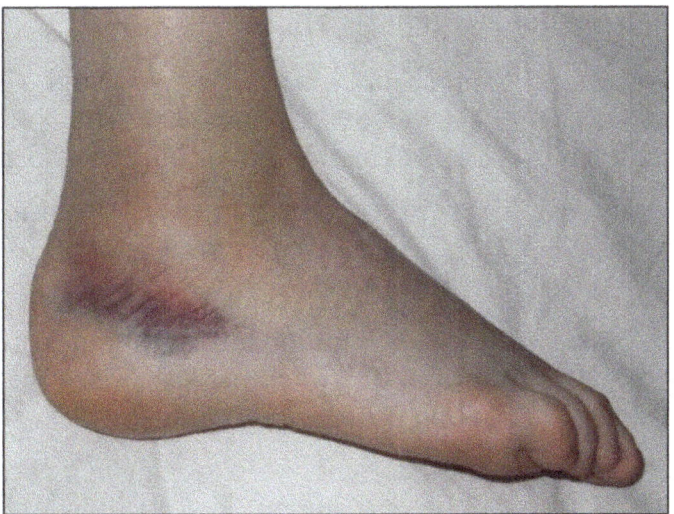

THIRD DEGREE SPRAIN

This is a complete rupture of the ligament, sometimes even with fracture of the bone. The patient is unable to mobilize and stabilize the joint. There is a lot of pain and bruising.

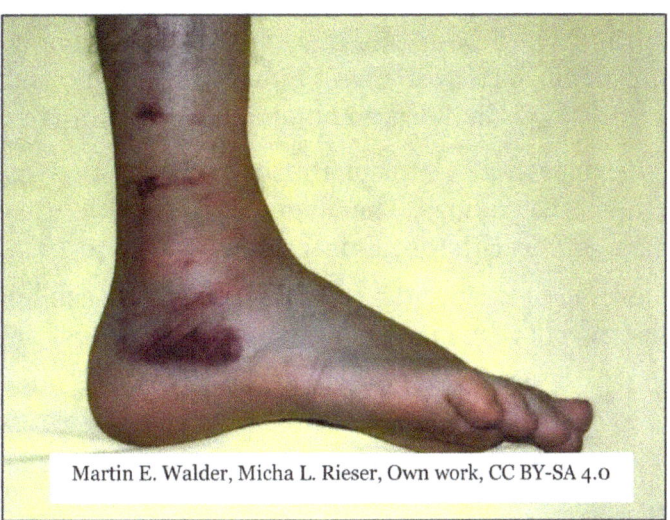

Martin E. Walder, Micha L. Rieser, Own work, CC BY-SA 4.0

Diagnosis

The sprain is easy to diagnose just by looking at it. It is a patient who has sprained a joint, most commonly the wrists and ankles, and has swelling and pain.

Try to gently move the joint so that you can appreciate the degree of resistance it presents. A very loose joint, which makes movements that are not proper for it, is an unstable joint and should be immobilized.

Treatment

Depending on the degree of the sprain, treatment will be either conservative or surgical. The general recommendations are to apply ice locally and to keep the limb elevated to improve the edema. Rosemary or chamomile infusions help to reduce the swelling of the soft tissues.

It is always a good idea to keep an ankle brace and a wrist brace on hand, which help support the joint and thus decrease swelling and discomfort. If you don't have one of these, you can use a normal bandage and make a firm dressing on the injured joint. Remember that the idea is to give stability.

An unstable, third-degree sprain should be evaluated by a specialist to decide if surgery is required. As long as it is not possible to seek help, it is necessary to immobilize that joint for at least four weeks. Ideally the immobilization would be with a brace, a splint, or a similar device.

If you don't have a splint, stabilization is done with homemade splints that you can make with strong boards, plates, or even with a ruler if you can't find anything else. Place the board under the limb you want to immobilize and secure the limb to that board with a bandage.

You want to give stability to the joint so that it does not keep moving in an errant way and does not have major damage. Obviously, this is not a definitive treatment, but it will help the patient feel better, avoid further damage, and rest the joint to improve swelling.

5. Fractures

A fracture is the loss of continuity in a bone, either partially or completely. Fractures are caused by various traumatic mechanisms, from sprains to direct blows, penetrating injuries and even shock waves in healthy bones, or low-intensity blows in diseased bones with osteoporosis or cancer.

Fractures are very painful because they damage the outer layer that covers the bone, called the periosteum, which contains the nerve endings. The diagnosis of the fracture can be intuited byanalyzing the mechanism of the trauma together with the clinical signs.

If you were not present at the time of the accident, it is important to ask how it happened, if he or she fell from a height or from their own height, and what the blow was against or what object hit the bone.

The fracture site will be seen to be enlarged by swelling and will be very painful and hypersensitive. If an x-ray is possible, that will make the definitive diagnosis.

When you encounter or suspect a fracture, make sure the person does not move the fractured limb. Try to immobilize the fracture with one of the techniques I mentioned earlier for sprains and dislocations.

In my country it is very common that when people have a fall or a trauma, they go to a specific place to get a special massage. These people (generally men) call themselves "sobadores" (rubbers).

They are supposed to have special techniques to heal any kind of ailment, similar to what Mr. Miyagi did in Karate Kid. Along with this rubbing, they say prayers to promote healing.

Sometimes people do get healed, but when there is a fracture, they only manage to make it worse because it can go from a simple fracture line to one with mobilization of both ends, which usually requires surgery. I think after reading this you might suspect that traumatologists hate "sobadores".

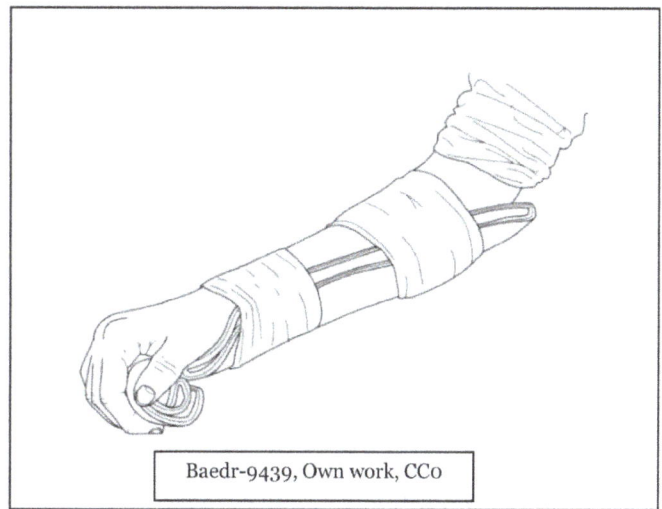
Baedr-9439, Own work, CC0

After immobilizing and relieving the pain with a painkiller, check their pulse to assess for vascular involvement. The pulse of the radial artery in the arm is easy to feel. It is located in the wrist on the same side as the thumb.

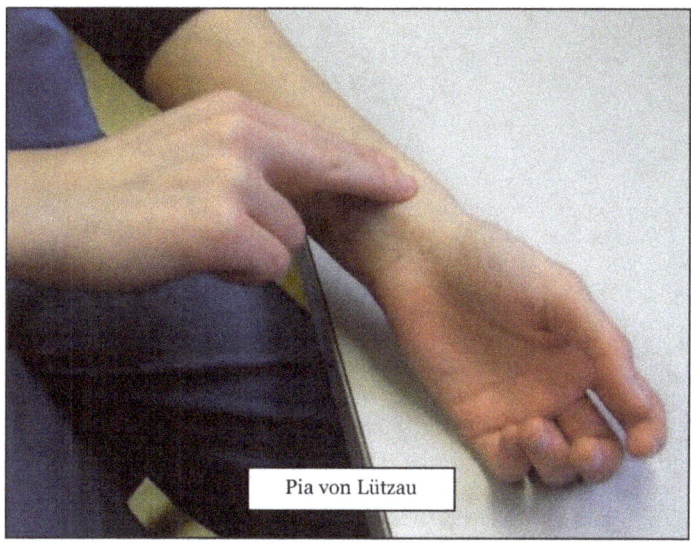
Pia von Lützau

In the foot, the pulse of the pedal artery will give you information about the circulation of the whole member. It is located in the central part of the metatarsal.

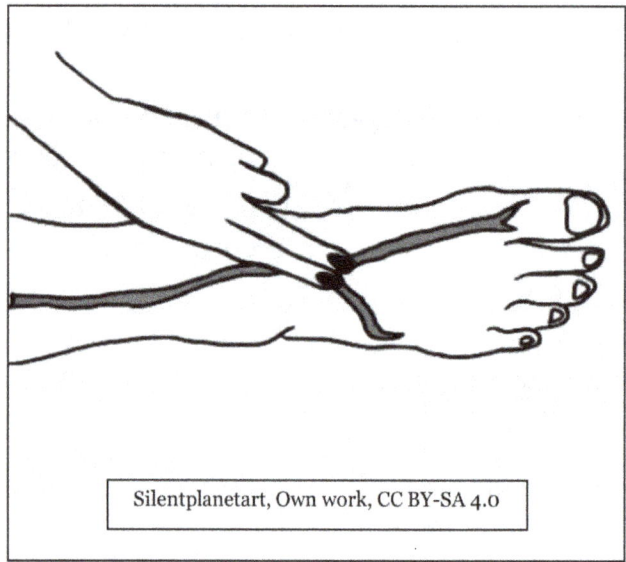

Silentplanetart, Own work, CC BY-SA 4.0

In the figure below, you can see all the places where you can find the pulse.

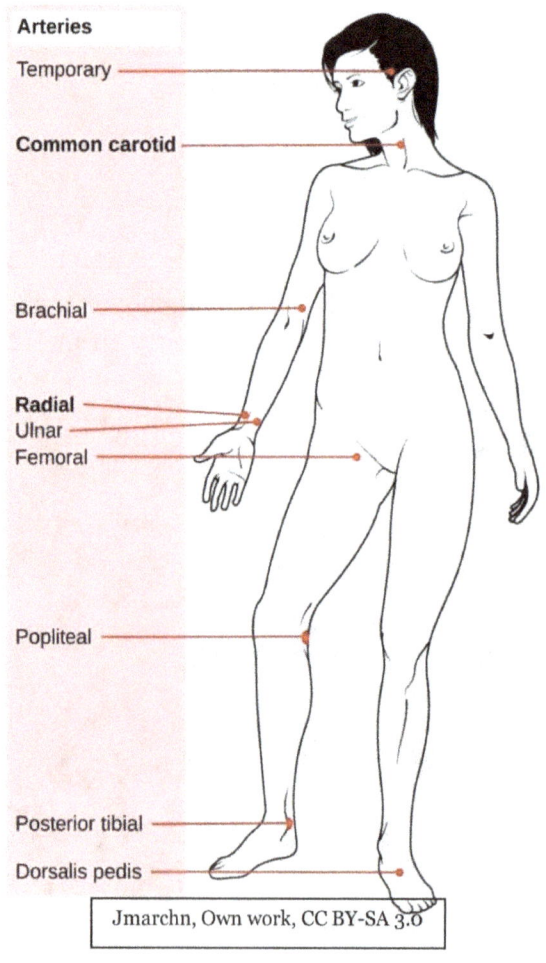

Jmarchn, Own work, CC BY-SA 3.0

CARDIOVASCULAR SYSTEM

The cardiovascular or circulatory system is a group of organs that allow the transport of blood for the nutrition of all the cells of the body. It consists of the heart, blood vessels (veins and arteries), and blood. Anatomy textbooks and atlases usually depict the arteries as red, the veins as blue, and the lymph vessels as green.

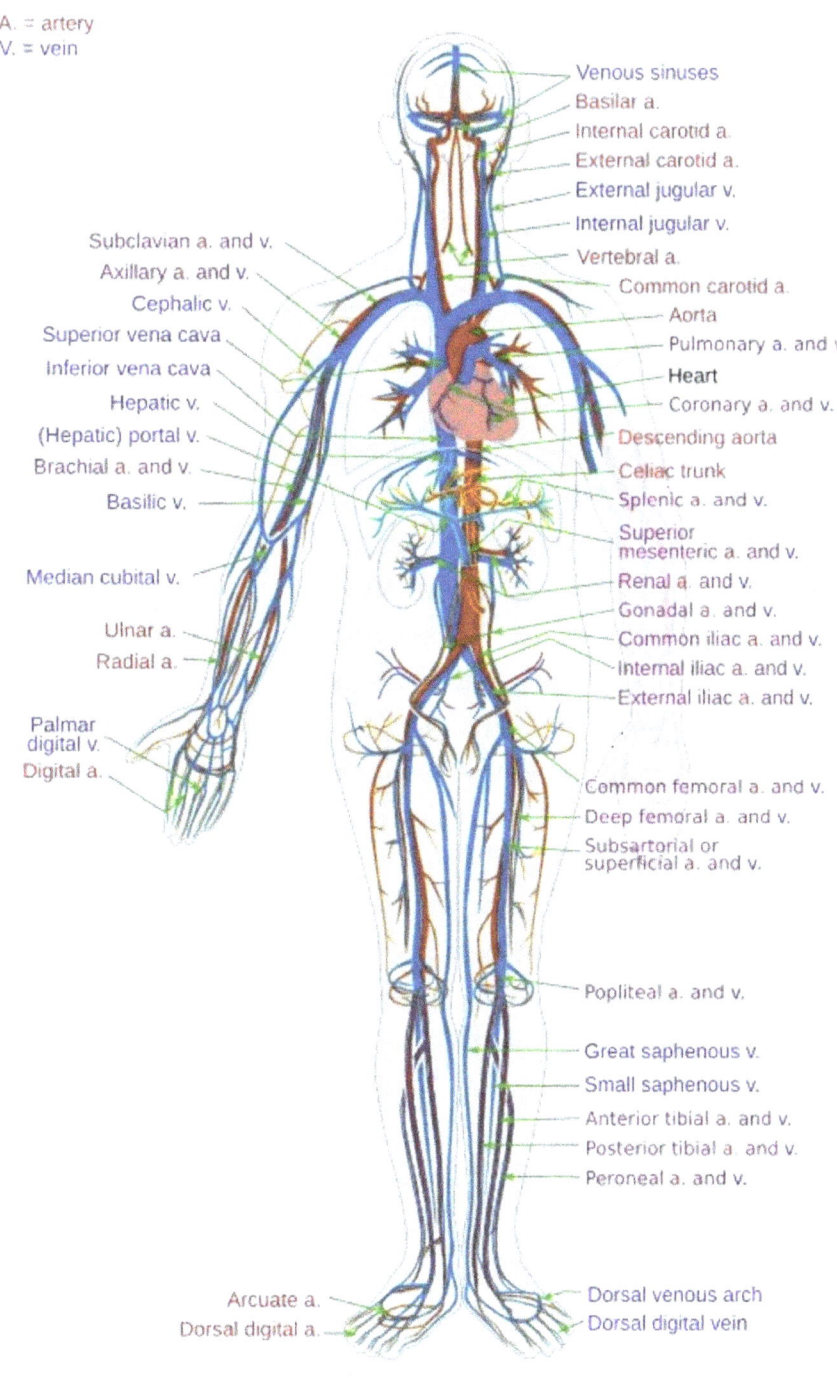

The **heart** is a hollow muscular organ that functions as a pump, carrying blood through two circulatory systems to the lungs and the rest of the body.

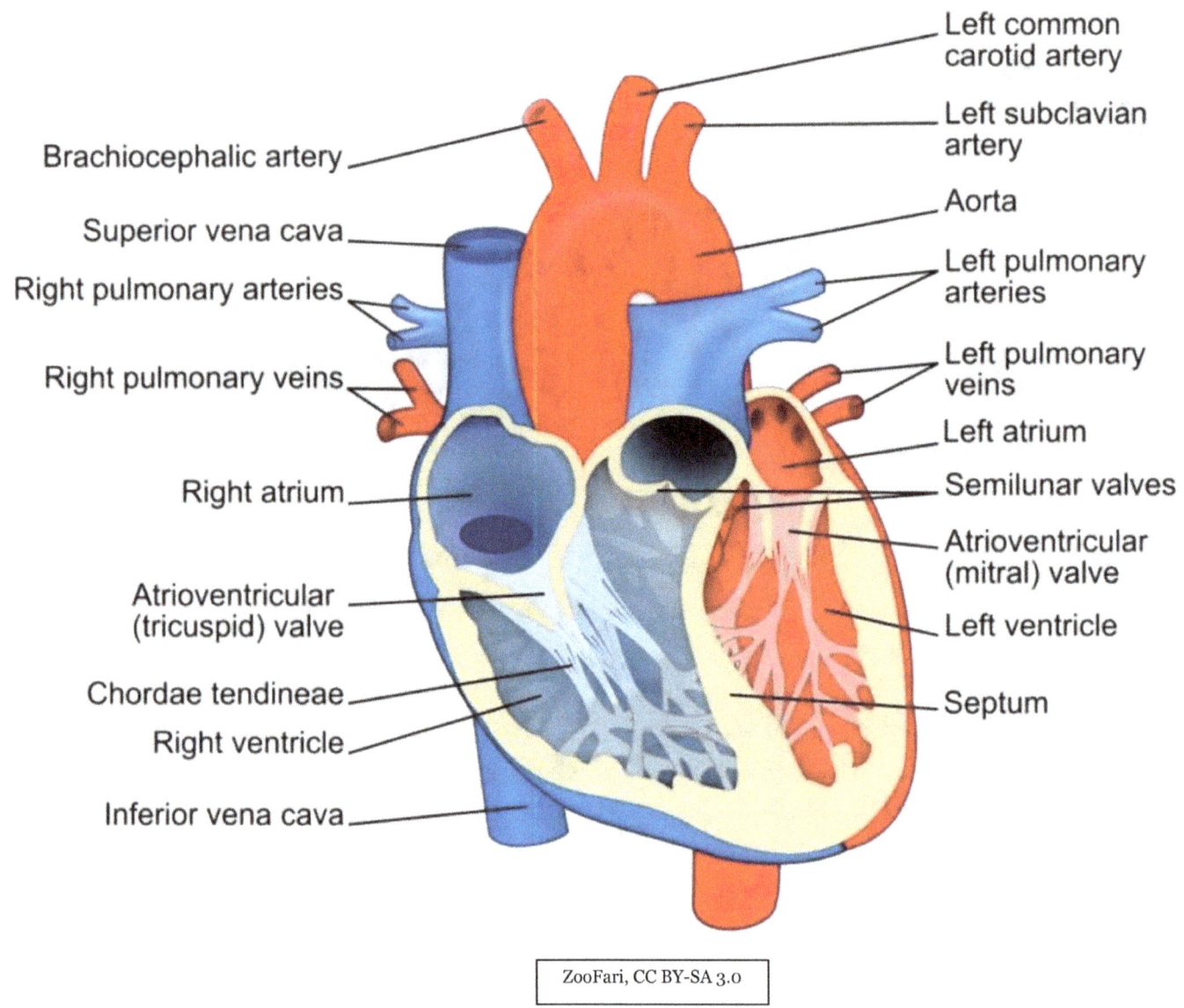

It is a vital organ, one of the most important in the entire body. Its injury is considered an absolute emergency, whether due to trauma or to changes in its structure, so you have to know how to manage a heart injury or failure to at least gain some time until help arrives.

The heart has a process of contracting and dilating its muscle that works automatically through electrical signals. Every heartbeat is the manifestation of that phenomenon.

A heartbeat pushes blood out of the heart and into the other organs. This happens at a rate of 80 times per minute, which is what we know as a heartbeat.

Since it is a mechanism that works with energy, any external change, such as an electrocution, can alter the heart's rhythm.

Arteries and **veins** are blood vessels that carry oxygenated and deoxygenated blood respectively. While the arteries are responsible for nourishing the organs, the veins collect the blood and return it to the pulmonary circulation to complete the oxygenation process and return it to the general circulation.

Pulmonary blood circulation, or minor blood circulation, is the process that occurs in the lungs through which blood without oxygen picks up oxygen ions and discards carbon dioxide ions, returning to the heart to enter the systemic circulation, or major circulation.

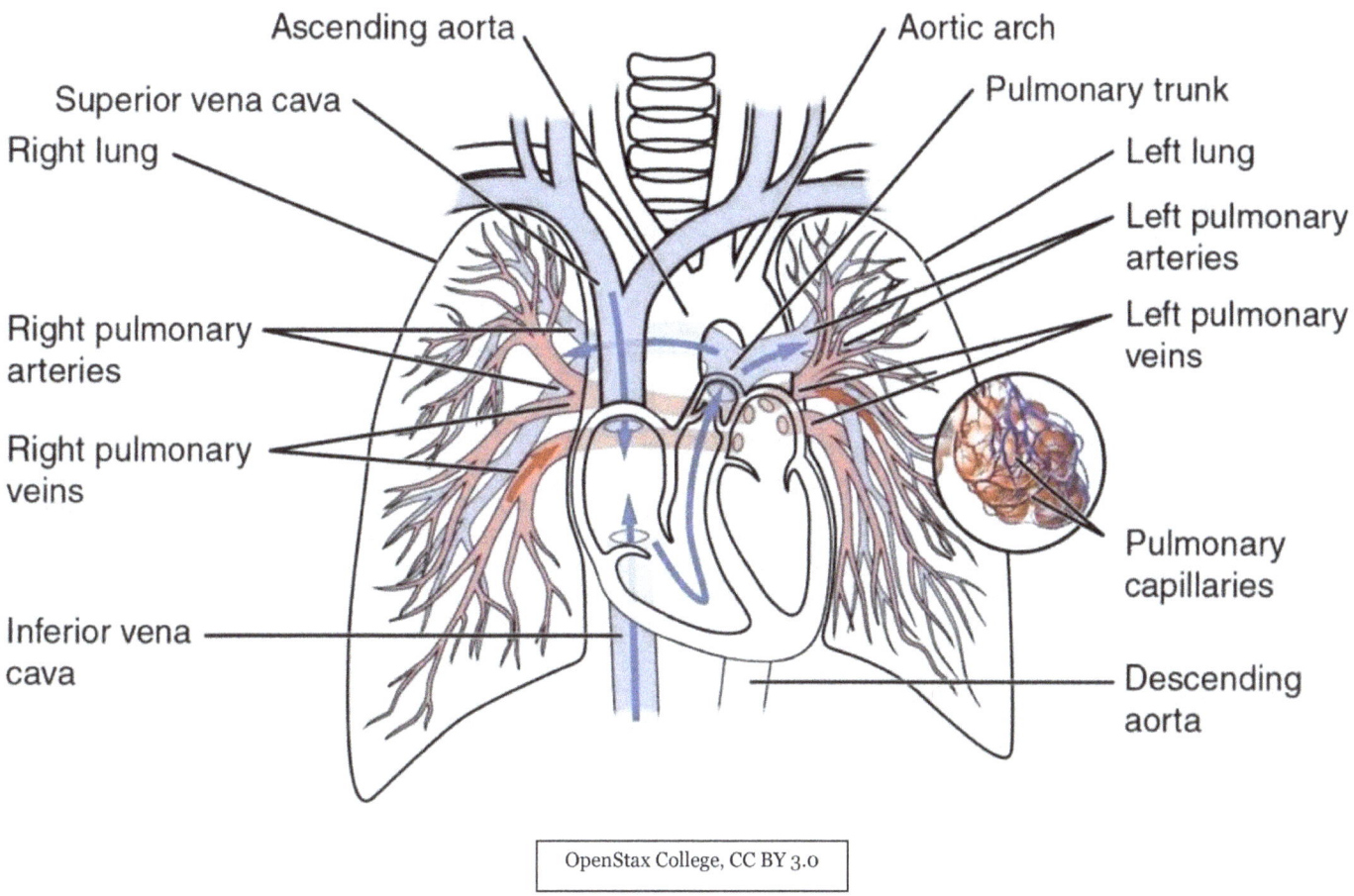

OpenStax College, CC BY 3.0

On the other hand, the systemic circulation is in charge of transporting the oxygenated blood from the heart to the rest of the body through the aorta and returning it through the vena cava.

Arteries are also muscular organs that must maintain tension in order to withstand the pressure with which blood passes through them. This is what we know as blood pressure. There is a contraction pressure and a relaxation pressure, so it is read as two numbers.

The normal pressure for an individual at rest is 120/80 mmHg +/- 10. When the person is agitated, exercising, or stressed, the pressure increases. On the other hand, if the person is resting or sleeping, it can be very low.

Blood pressure is a parameter that helps us identify many disorders of the vascular system. If the person is chronically hypertensive, we can know that their kidneys are suffering as well as their eyes since these pressure changes alter the most sensitive organs.

In addition, the arteries enter a state of stress due to the amount of force they exert and can break or collapse, generating serious problems such as cerebrovascular disease or myocardial infarction.

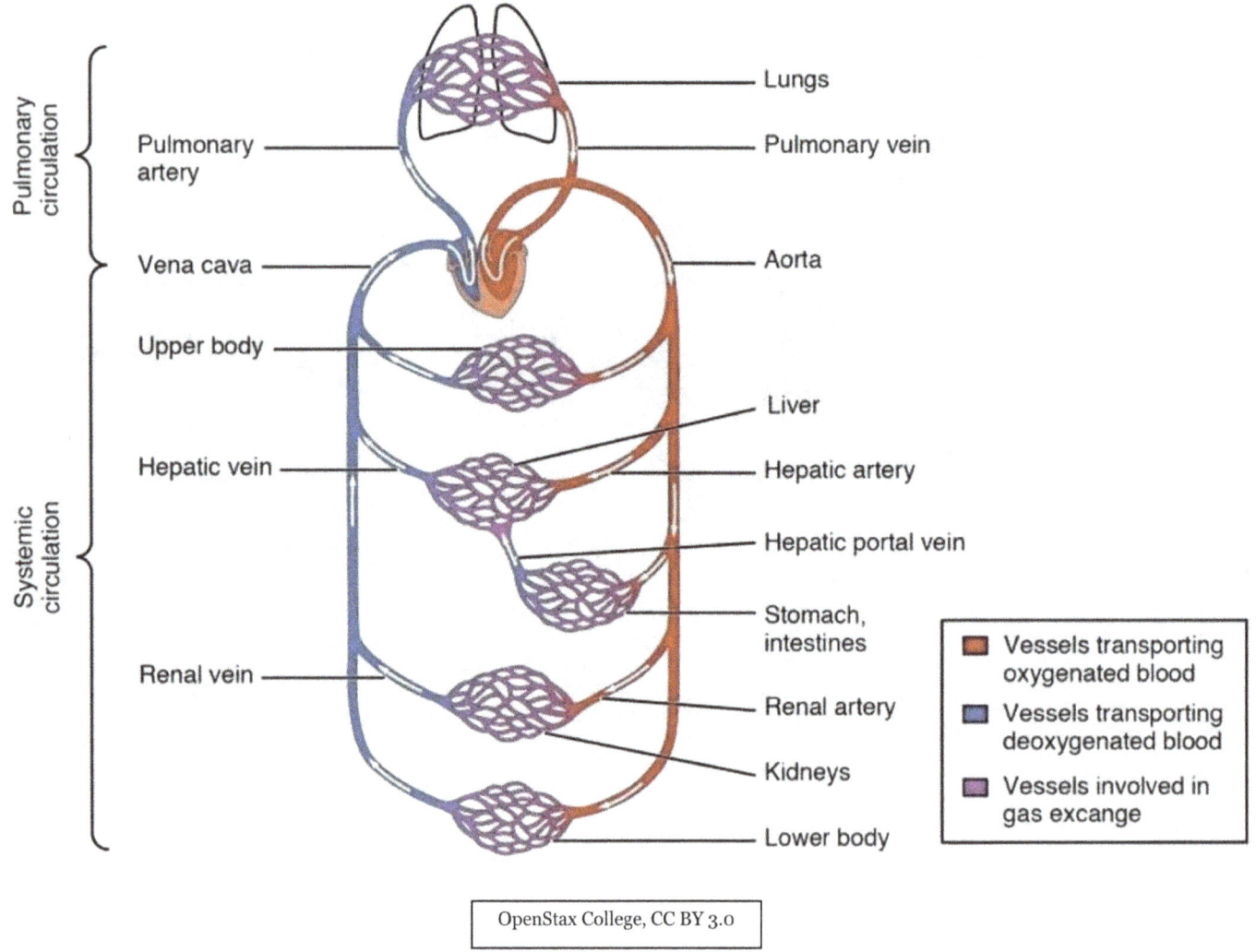

OpenStax College, CC BY 3.0

The physical assessment of the cardiovascular system begins with the identification of the pulse and blood pressure.

A blood pressure monitor is one of the best investments you can make. I have two at home, and I gave one to my parents since they are both hypertensive. Some monitors also mark the heart rate although I rely more on measuring it manually.

HOW DO I MEASURE MY PULSE AND BLOOD PRESSURE?

The most common way to take a pulse is at the wrist through the radial artery pulse, which is one inch from the wrist joint, following the line of the thumb. The pulse should be taken with the index and middle fingers, not the thumb, as the thumb receives waves from the pulse and can give an altered rate. Although this is the most common way, there are many other places where a person's pulse can be measured.

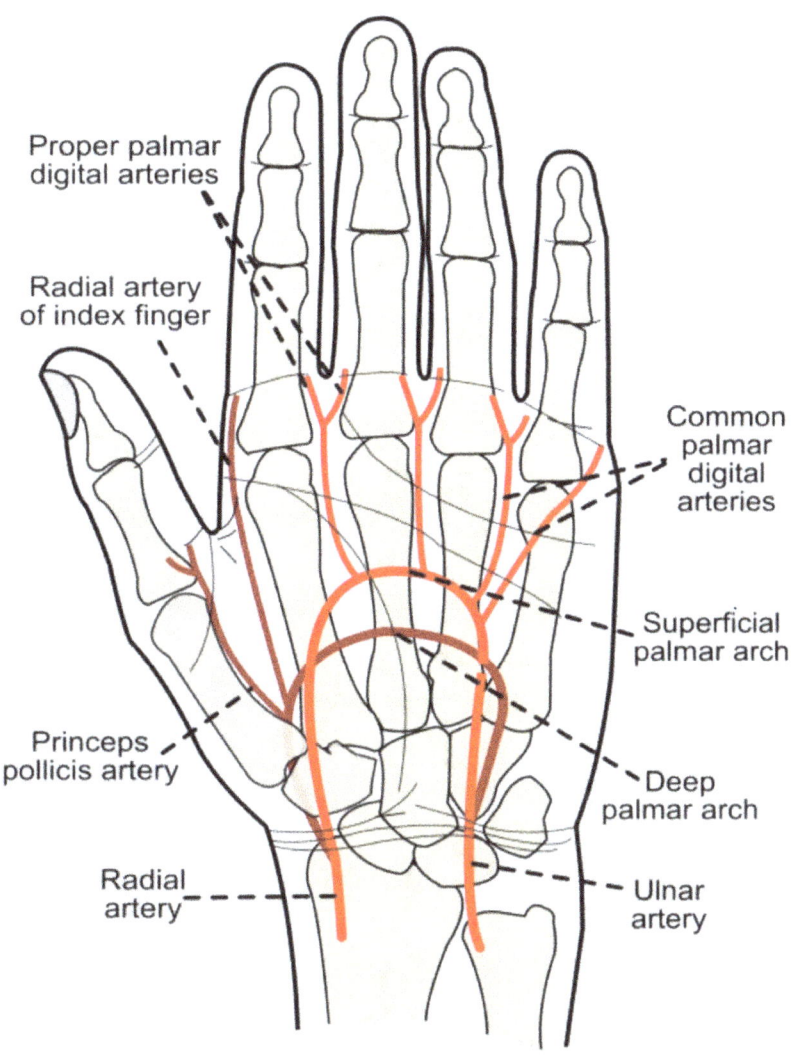

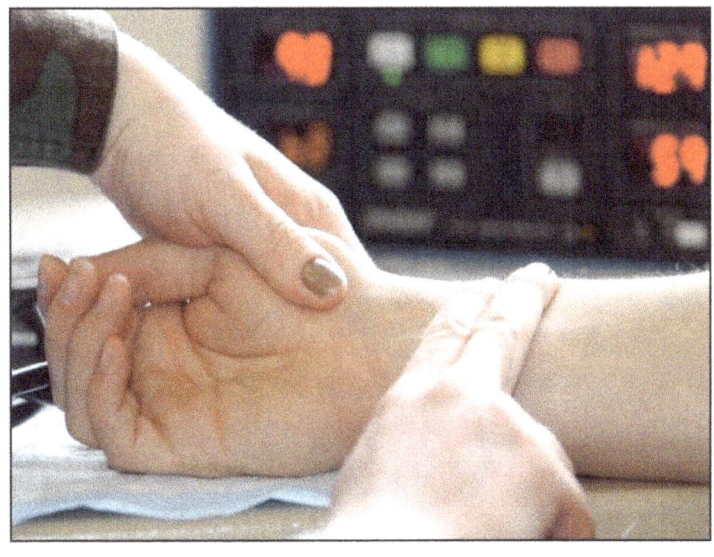

There are situations where you will not be able to take a radial pulse, for example in very obese people, burned arms, and amputees, among others.

In addition, sometimes you will have to take other pulses not only to count the rate but also to evaluate the quality of the circulation in that site. In the following figure, you can see the places on the body where you find superficial arteries in order to feel a person's pulse.

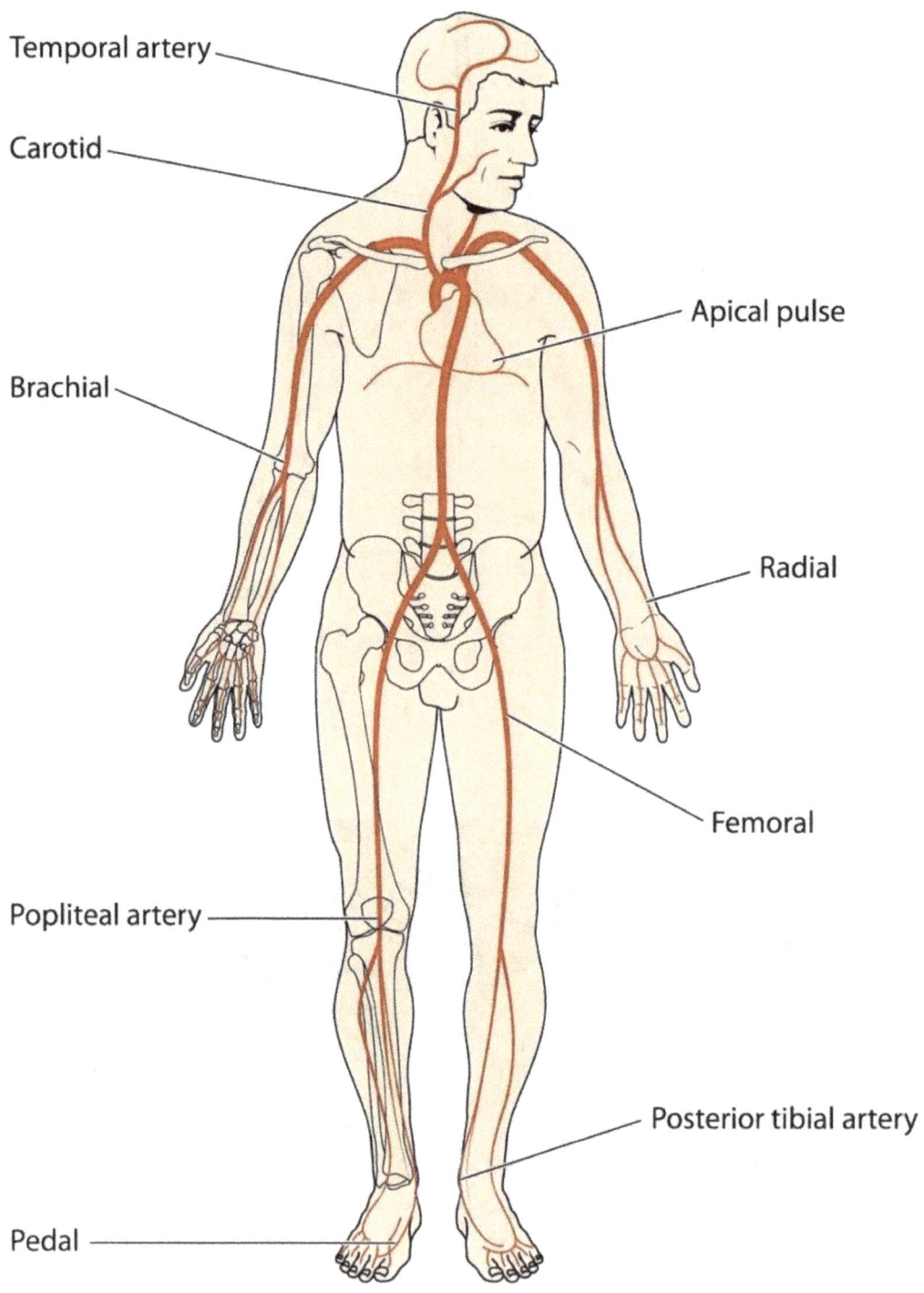

Blood pressure is the pressure that blood exerts on the arteries that makes them generate tension to maintain an adequate circulatory flow. At the doctor's office, you will probably have your blood pressure measured with a sphygmomanometer, which is a hand-held device for measuring blood pressure. It requires some training to use.

That is why at home, the simplest and most practical thing is to have a digital pressure monitor.

Physical activity alters blood pressure values, so before measuring, it is important that the person is kept at rest for 10 minutes. The pressure is taken with the patient sitting halfway down, and the arm resting on a surface so that it is at the same level as the heart.

If the gauge is a wrist gauge, you must ensure that your hand is at heart level.

To measure the tension in the arm, you must be shirtless or wearing short sleeves. The idea is that you don't have to roll up your sleeves so they are tight on your arm.

The pouf should be positioned one inch above the crease of the elbow without tightening it or leaving it too loose as this can alter the result. The hose is aligned with the brachial artery, which runs through the middle of the elbow crease. This way the results will be most accurate.

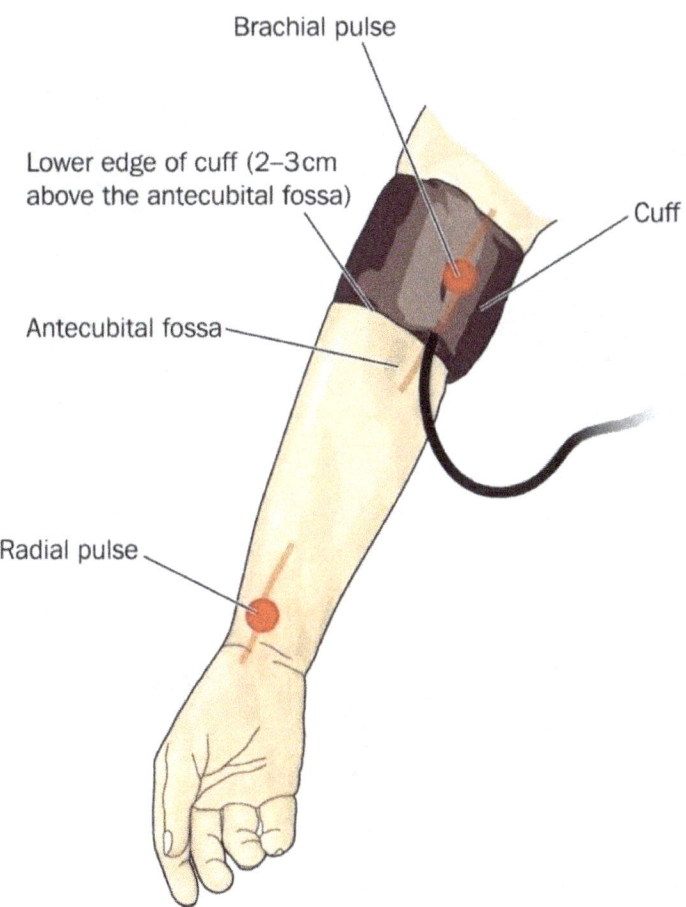

It is appropriate to take several pressure readings during the day so that you can see if the pressure fluctuates or if there are times when high-pressure peaks occur.

It is very important to note the result with the date and time. All this information will be useful in an emergency. Remember that the more information you have to provide, the better.

MEASURING BLOOD PRESSURE WITHOUT EQUIPMENT

You should know that without the proper equipment, you can only make a rough estimate of the blood pressure. Nowadays there are phone applications that can calculate your pressure. They are all inaccurate, but this is a tool that eventually will become part of everyday use.

Another method is even more inaccurate than the previous one, but as I said before, it is important to know since it is a guide that you can take into account in an emergency. This measurement is done with three pulses: the carotid, the radial. and the femoral.

The carotid pulse is taken in the neck, on the sides of the larynx, where the artery makes its most superficial route. When you feel a clear pulse without pressing your fingers on the artery, it means that your diastolic blood pressure is above 60 mmHg.

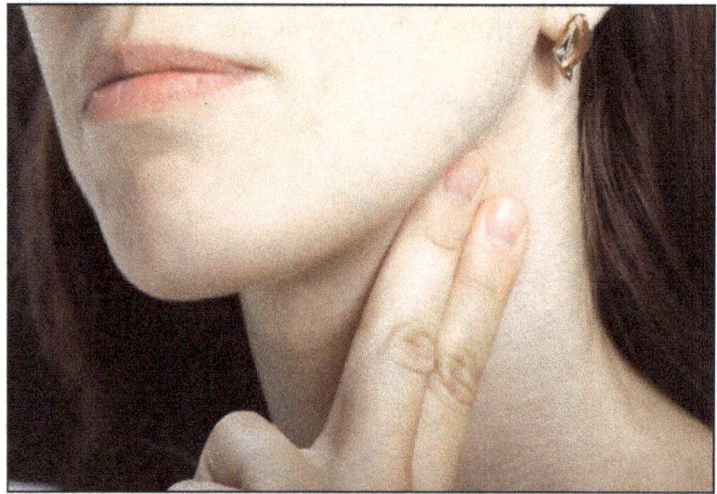

The radial pulse is then taken using the technique explained above. Palpation of this pulse means that you have a systolic blood pressure of at least 80 mmHg.

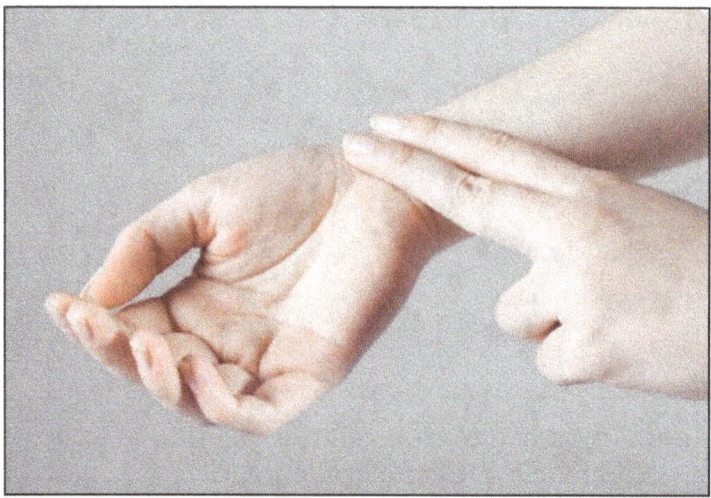

Finally, the femoral pulse is palpated, in the groin. When this pulse is palpable, the patient has blood pressure of approximately 70 mmHg.

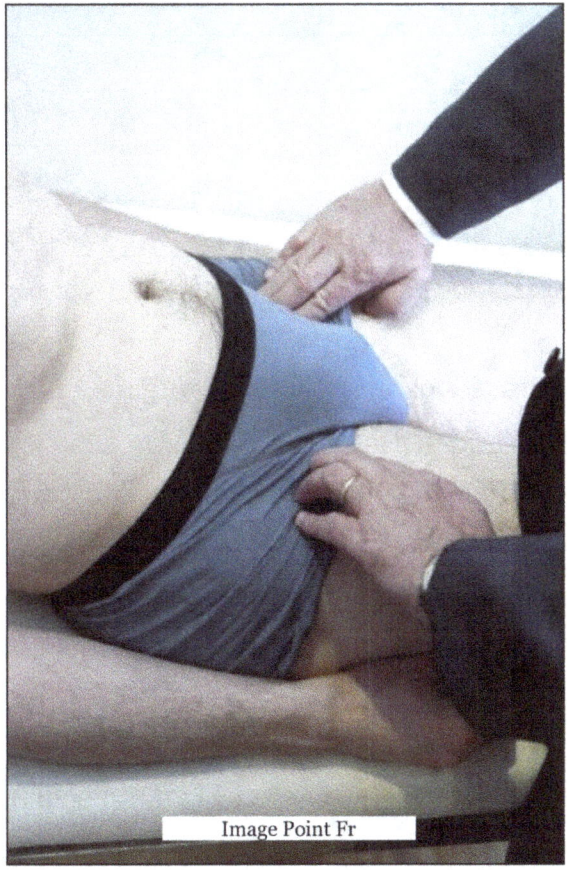

If these three pulses can be clearly felt without any effort, that person has acceptable blood pressure. When a strong pulse is felt and hits the fingers, the blood pressure is elevated. Conversely, when it cannot be felt, it means low blood pressure. This test should be correlated with the rest of the patient's symptoms.

Remember that this is a very basic test that only gives you a rough reference of the blood pressure but not enough to take a drug treatment.

1. High Blood Pressure

High blood pressure could be a chronic condition characterized by a sustained increase in vessel pressure over time. Its importance lies in the fact that many times by the time it is diagnosed, there has already been irreparable damage to various tissues as it presents very few or no symptoms at all in its early stages. That is why it is called the "Silent Killer."

The diagnosis of hypertension or high blood pressure is made by measuring blood pressure for seven consecutive days, twice a day at the same time. If the pressure is found to be high all or most days, the patient is diagnosed with the condition.

International Society of Hypertension: Global Hypertension Practice Guidelines (2020)

Category	Systolic, mmHg	Diastolic, mmHg
HYPOTENSION	<90	<60
NORMAL	<130	<85
HIGH NORMAL	130-139	85-89
Grade 1 HYPERTENSION	140-159	90-99
Grade 2 HYPERTENSION	>160	>100

Left untreated, high blood pressure causes damage to various organs, and if it is not diagnosed in time, the damage may be irreparable.

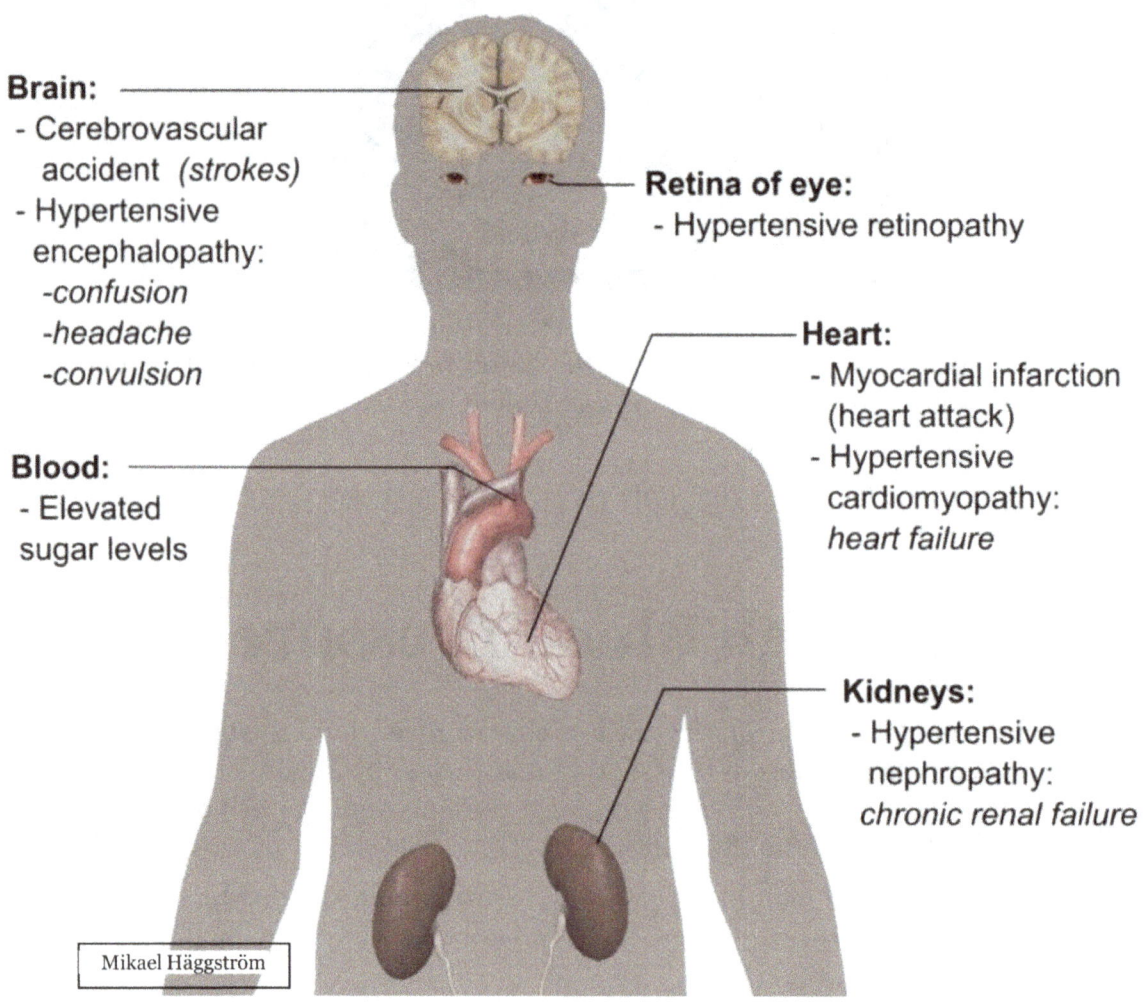

Treatment

The pharmacological treatment of hypertension is delicate and is indicated by a specialist according to the type of hypertension and the damage that occurs. Usually an antihypertensive is indicated, and thisis combined with diuretics, which are drugs that increase urination.

In this section, I want to focus on natural treatment as there are many ways to lower blood pressure with infusions and dietary changes. From the many scientific studies that have been done, evidence has been found that they work very well to decrease high blood pressure.

At no time do I seek to replace the medications that must be taken for high blood pressure. I am simply interested in sharing all these remedies, some learned in Amazonas and others from patients' comments, who always keep me informed of the classic popular medications I don't know about.

Natural Management of High Blood Pressure

Antihypertensives are relatively new agents, developed only in the 20th century. However, hypertension as a disease was described by Al-Akhawayni Bukhari, a 10th century Persian physician who made important contributions to modern medicine.

His book, *Student's Handbook of Medicine*, the oldest document of Iranian traditional medicine, detailsa disease with symptoms similar to those of high blood pressure. It was attributed to an overload of blood in the body. The treatments proposed at that time resembled the current ones, suggesting changes in lifestyle, physical activity, and the consumption of some foods that currently have been shown to have beneficial effects on this disease.

What was done in the 10th century and is still in practice today?

  1. *Leeches*

Although it is not the most widely used treatment nowadays, there are still populations that use leechesas a medical tool. They are widely used in fractures and in traumas that are considered serious for their analgesic, anti-inflammatory, and anticoagulant properties in addition to the number of enzymes foundin their saliva.

They are used for high blood pressure because they decrease the amount of blood circulating so that the arteries do not need to exert as much pressure.

In addition to leeches, bleeding therapies were used by breaking a blood vessel and allowing it to bleedin a controlled manner until the treatment was considered to be effective.

Leeches are not uncommon in modern medicine; for some time, they were used as a means of securing reimplants of limbs, especially hands and fingers. In Amazonas, among the indigenous people, this practice exists for many purposes, such as improving the heaviness of legs due to varicose veins and cleansing those who suffer from bad temper or bad luck.

  2. *Bitter Tea*

Bitter tea is an infusion prepared with a flower called Jamaica (Hibiscus sabdariffa), which is widely used in natural medicine for its healing, anti-inflammatory and relaxing properties. Its benefits have been observed for a long time as to how it controls high blood pressure, which has led to scientific studies demonstrating its usefulness.

It can be taken cold or hot; it has a very particular taste that some will find very acidic, but it can be sweetened and looks fantastic. In addition to its use for high blood pressure, it is a natural diuretic, so it helps with fluid retention, relieves inflammation, and helps with sleep because it is a powerful relaxant.

3. Garlic

Garlic is used both as a spread and as a poultice or included in food as an anti-inflammatory, vasodilator, and antiseptic. In the case of high blood pressure, its dilating effect on blood vessels helps to lower it by up to 10 mmHg. I have heard many strange ways to consume garlic. The strangest one someone told me about was garlic tea. According to this patient, this infusion tastes very bad, but its healing properties are worth it. She sweetens it with honey to mitigate the strong taste.

There are those who eat garlic cloves raw, and others who eat it roasted; I can say from experience that it is delicious that way. There are also garlic capsules for those who cannot stand the taste or the breath but want to receive the benefits.

It is not recommended in the case of bleeding or stroke because it seems to have an anticoagulant effect. In fact, this warning is specified in Al-Akhawayni Bukhari's 10th century handbook.

My patient's garlic tea recipe

You will need 4 cloves of garlic, 2 cups of water, 1 tablespoon honey, and lemon (optional). Peel and cut the garlic cloves in half. Bring the water to a boil with the garlic cloves. Let it cook for 7 minutes, turn off the heat, and add the honey and lemon, if desired. You can consume it cold or hot up to 3 cups a day.

4. Dark Chocolate

Cocoa is a typical product of my country with a lot of history. From the times when it was mixed with tobacco and smoked to the chocolate bar we know today, cocoa has been used for medicinal purposes for quite some time.

Dark chocolate has at least 70% cocoa. This ensures that you can enjoy the chocolate bar and all the medicinal benefits of cocoa as well.

This product is rich in flavanol, a natural chemical that increases the release of nitric oxide and dilates the blood vessels, decreasing blood pressure. A one-ounce serving of dark chocolate is recommended daily to take advantage of the antihypertensive effects.

Venezuelan cocoa is some of the best in the world in terms of quality. There are many cocoa-producing areas, mostly coastal zones, where they sell unusual cocoa products, such as cocoa paste, wine, cream punch, cocoa shell tea, body creams, bath splash, bath salts, scrub, handmade soaps, and special syrups for different ailments.

Other foods, such as oats, almonds, berries, and potassium-rich fruits such as bananas and tomatoes, have good results in the natural treatment of hypertension, although there is no scientific evidence for the products listed above.

Preventing Hypertension and Keeping Blood Pressure Low

Some beneficial lifestyle changes are included in the treatment and prevention of hypertension.

Regular physical activity helps lower the resting heart rate, which benefits cardiovascular health. I recommend one hour of gentle exercise, 40 minutes of moderate activity, or 30 minutes of vigorous activity daily.

Quitting smoking is one of the most important recommendations for improving the condition of the cardiovascular system. Smoking produces a vasoconstrictive effect and affects the circulation in the small arteries, even clogging them.

If you are overweight, getting to an appropriate weight is very beneficial for cardiovascular health.

Losing weight is not just a matter of aesthetics. Obesity brings problems to many systems, including circulatory problems due to the accumulation of atheroma plaques. It also increases the risk of heart disease. It is important to maintain an adequate body mass index (BMI). The BMI is calculated with the formula *weight (kg) / height (meters) ²*. A BMI below 25 kg/m² is normal.

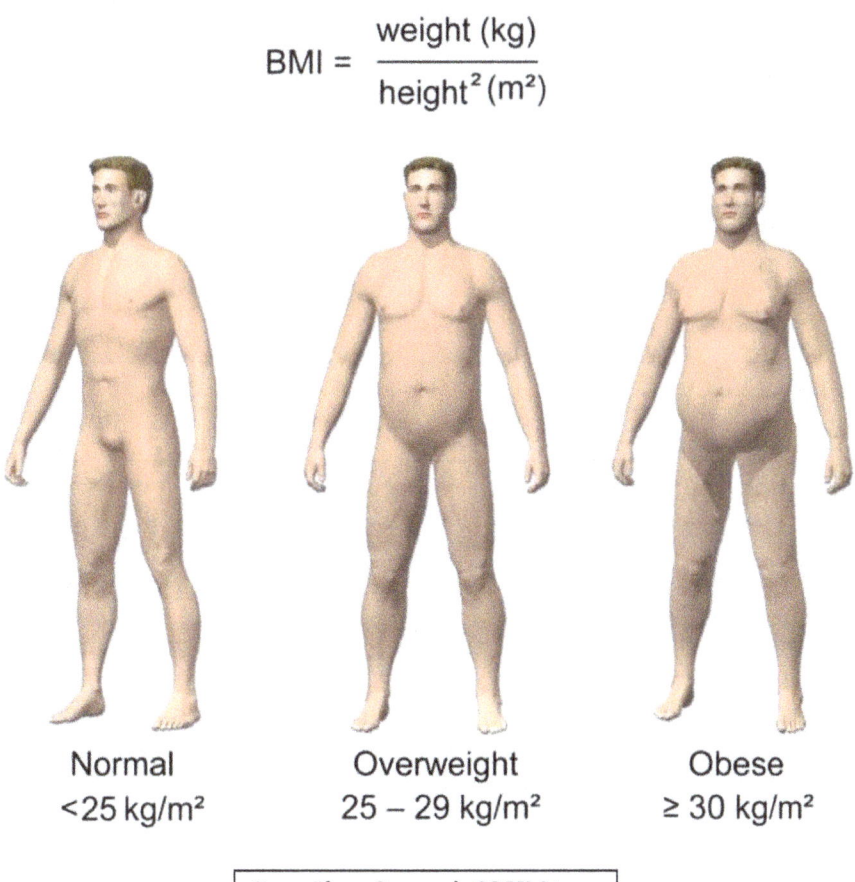

Bruce Blaus, Own work, CC BY-SA 4.0

Given the alarming levels of obesity worldwide, the terms "morbid obesity" for people with a BMI greater than 40 kg/m2 and "super obese" for people with a BMI greater than 50 kg/m2 have been included.

Whether an overweight or obese person loses weight naturally or through bariatric surgery, the benefits at the metabolic level are visible, especially its effect on hypertension.

Improving stress levels through meditation, exercise, or yoga helps maintain proper blood pressure. Eating a balanced diet with sufficient sources of protein and fat, such as avocado and salmon, has the same effect.

Remember that the only way to diagnose increased blood pressure is by measurement. Otherwise, it is a condition that has no major symptoms, so it can be present for many years without manifesting itself and the first symptoms can be serious, irreversible damage.

2. Cardiovascular Emergencies

Chest Pain

Chest pain is a warning sign because it can mean a life-threatening situation, such as a heart attack. However, there are many entities that cause chest pain, both cardiac and non-cardiac.

Non-cardiac causes include gastrointestinal, pulmonary, bone, and muscle causes. Also, infections such as herpes zoster (shingles) cause pain from the passage of the nerve that is infected and can be a cause of chest pain.

Characteristics of Chest Pain	Diagnosis
• Starts after eating, bringing up food or bitter-tasting fluids • Feeling full and bloated	*Gastro-esophageal reflux (GERD)*
• Starts after chest injury or chest exercise • Feels better when resting the muscle	*Chest sprain or strain*
• Triggered by worries or a stressful situation • Heartbeat gets faster • Sweating • Dizziness	*Anxiety* *Panic attack*
• Gets worse when you breathe in and out • Coughing up yellow or green mucus • High temperature	*Pneumonia*
• Tingling feeling on skin • Skin rash appears that turns into blisters	*Shingles*

ENDOCRINE SYSTEM

The endocrine system is an organized mechanism of glands that produce and secrete chemical substances named hormones, which are used for different metabolic processes in the body.

It is comparable to the nervous system in the sense that the former uses nerve impulses to carry out its functions and the latter uses hormonal action. Some glands have ducts through which they release their secretions, such as the salivary glands. These are called exocrine glands. On the other hand, endocrine glands are those that have their product travel through the circulation and selectively find its target organs.

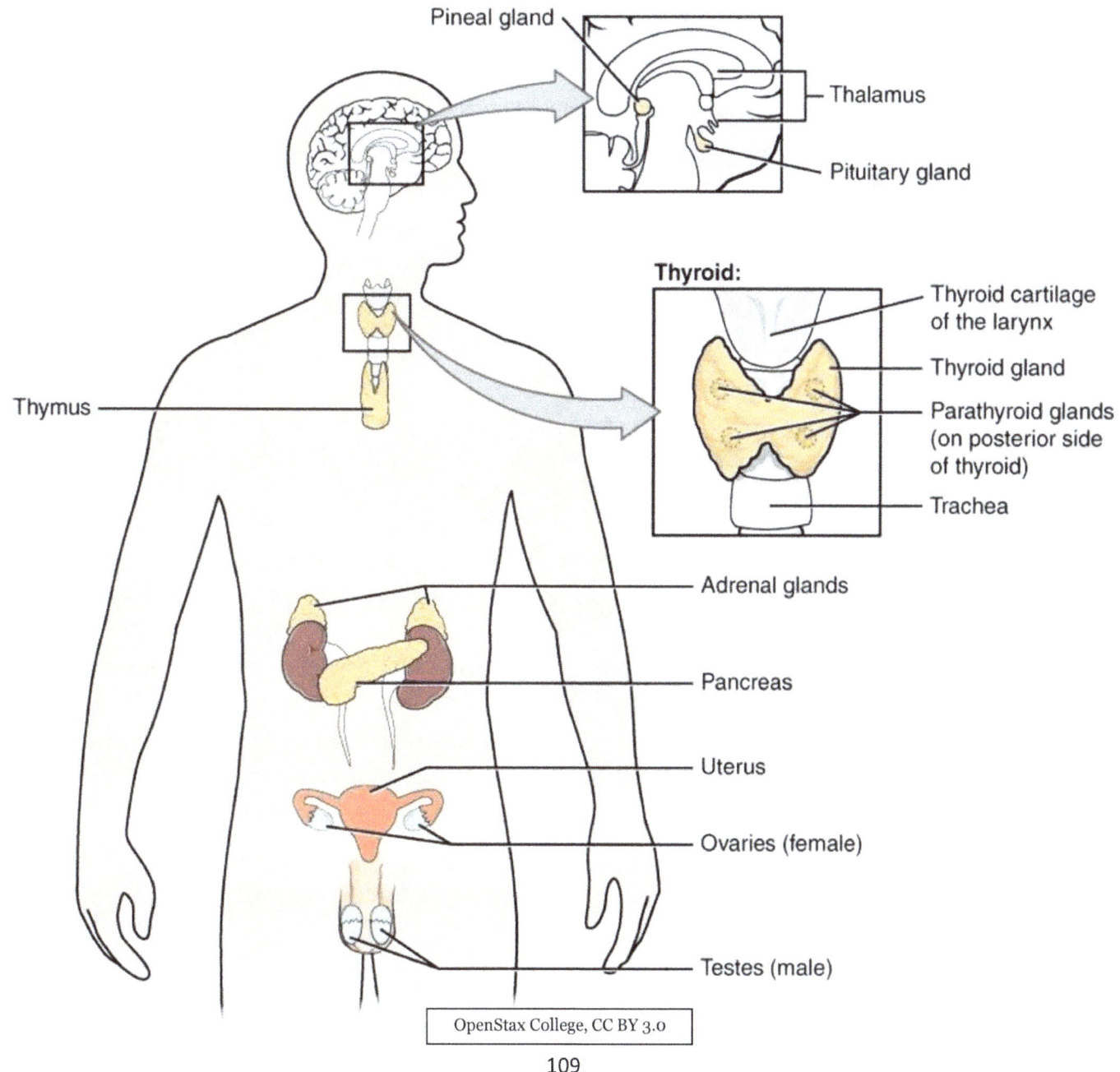

OpenStax College, CC BY 3.0

The endocrine system, through hormones, regulates many important metabolic processes. Some of its functions are:

- Growth and development
- Sexual function and reproduction
- Heart rate
- Blood pressure
- Appetite
- Sleeping and waking cycles
- Body temperature

The endocrine system regulates its functions through feedback loops. This means that a hormone that stimulates the secretion of a product stops being produced as soon as that product is in circulation in sufficient quantity.

Once the amount decreases, the hormone production will be activated again.

By the time any hormonal imbalance occurs, the symptoms are noticeable, and treatment is required to regulate the secretion and use of the hormones. This treatment is sometimes medical and sometimes surgical.

In the figures below, you can see the hormones produced by each of the body's endocrine glands.

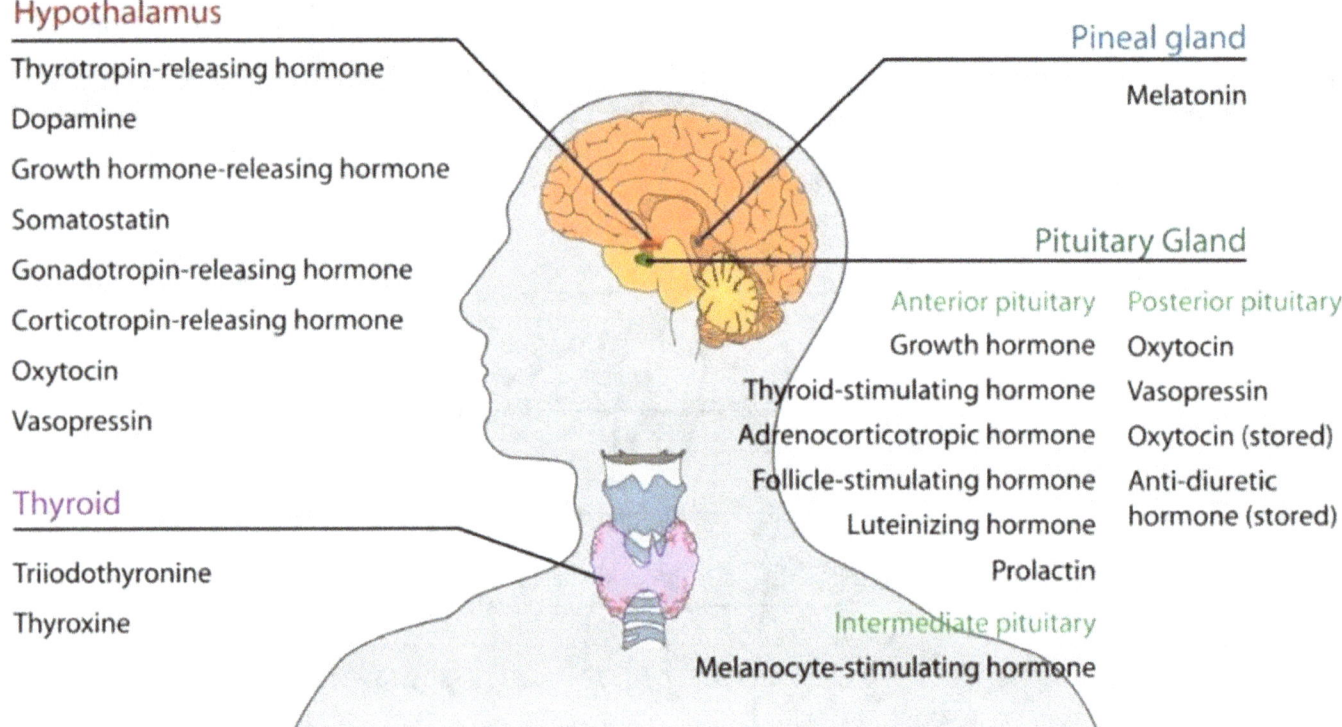

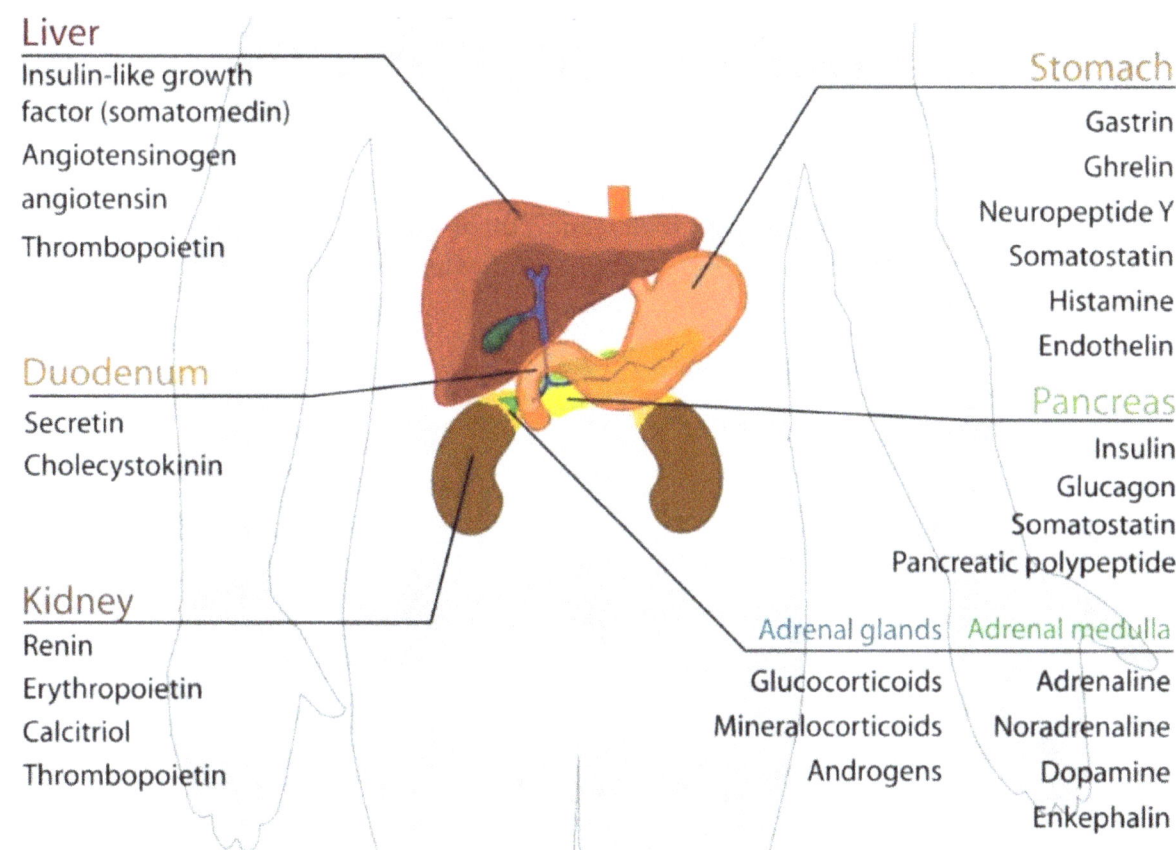

Liver
Insulin-like growth factor (somatomedin)
Angiotensinogen
angiotensin
Thrombopoietin

Duodenum
Secretin
Cholecystokinin

Kidney
Renin
Erythropoietin
Calcitriol
Thrombopoietin

Stomach
Gastrin
Ghrelin
Neuropeptide Y
Somatostatin
Histamine
Endothelin

Pancreas
Insulin
Glucagon
Somatostatin
Pancreatic polypeptide

Adrenal glands
Glucocorticoids
Mineralocorticoids
Androgens

Adrenal medulla
Adrenaline
Noradrenaline
Dopamine
Enkephalin

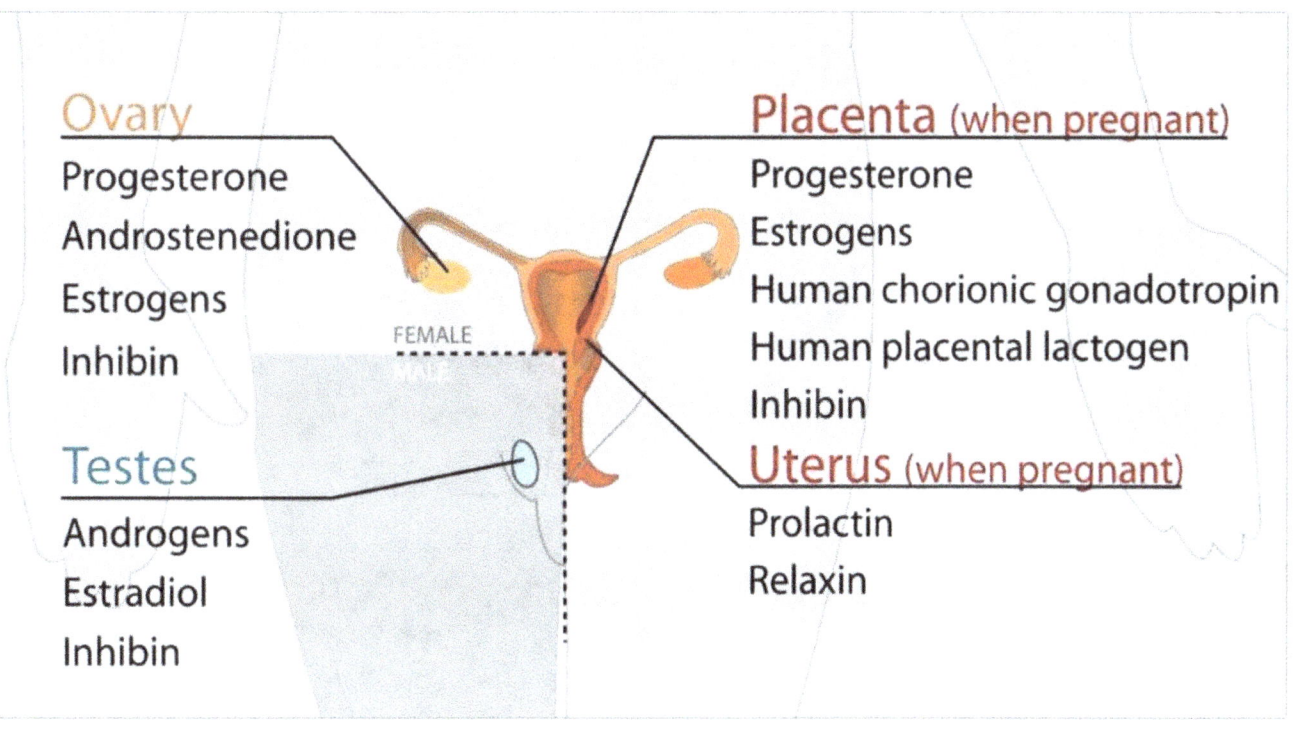

Ovary
Progesterone
Androstenedione
Estrogens
Inhibin

Testes
Androgens
Estradiol
Inhibin

Placenta (when pregnant)
Progesterone
Estrogens
Human chorionic gonadotropin
Human placental lactogen
Inhibin

Uterus (when pregnant)
Prolactin
Relaxin

1. Pancreas: Diabetes Mellitus Types 1 and 2

The pancreas is an organ of the digestive system located in the upper abdomen, behind the stomach. It is in direct communication with the duodenum through a duct where it discharges digestive enzymes. It also has functions in the internal metabolism of glucose.

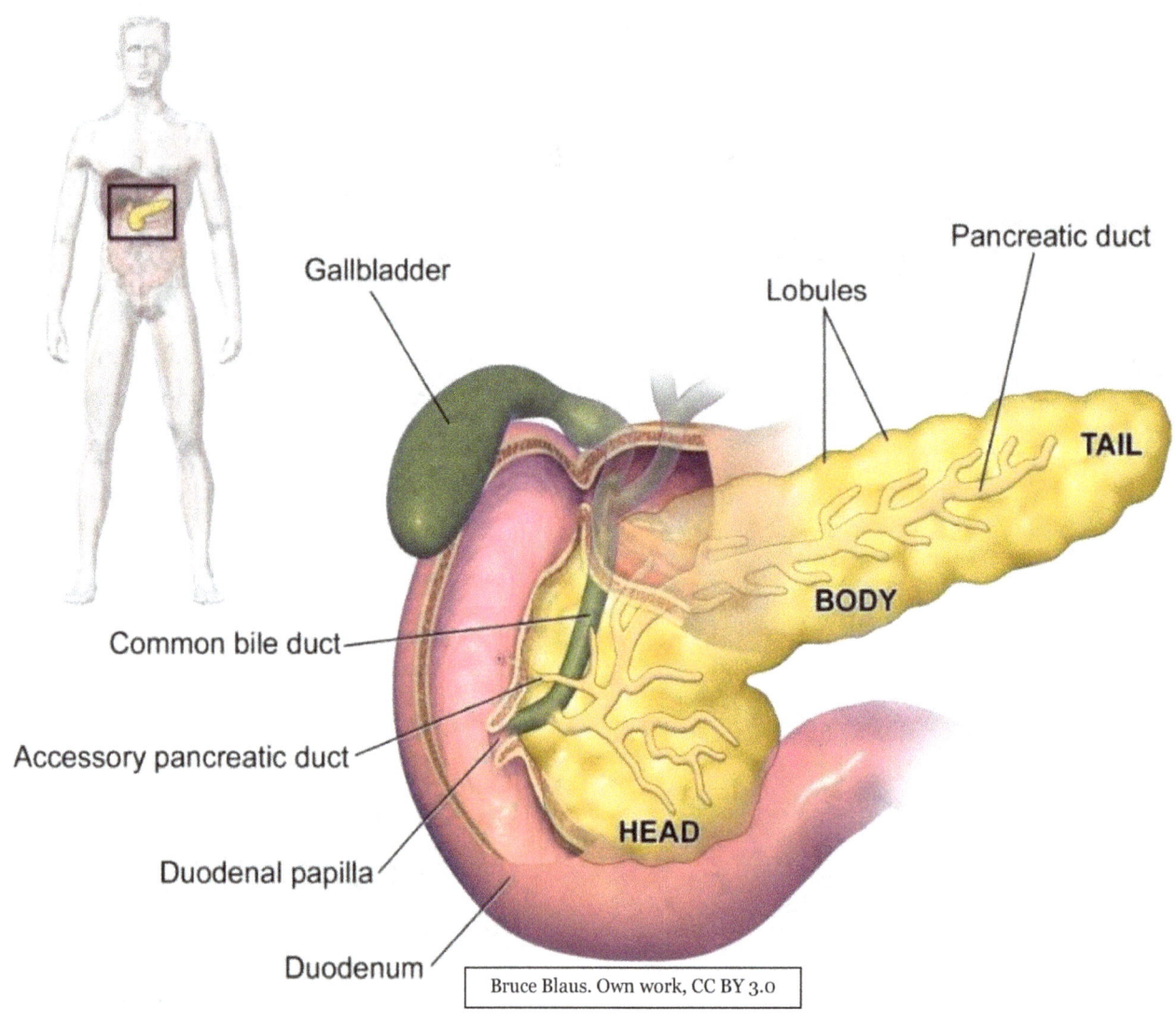

Bruce Blaus. Own work, CC BY 3.0

The pancreas regulates the amount of glucose in the blood through the release of various hormones, with insulin being the most important in the process. The pancreas is said to be an organ with both exocrine and endocrine function.

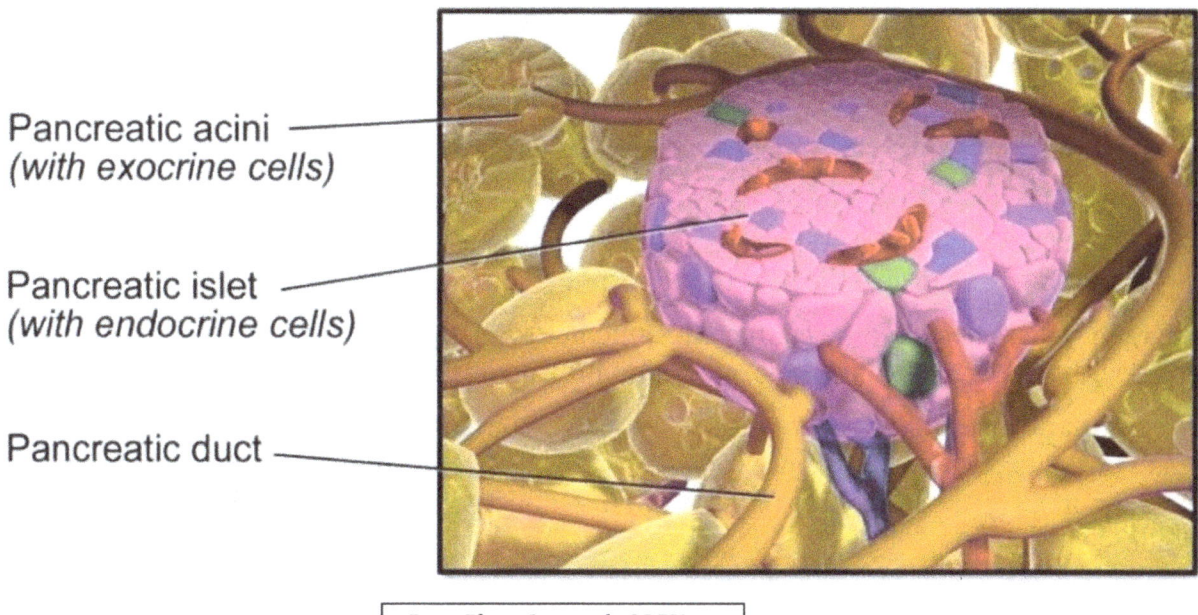

Bruce Blaus. Own work, CC BY 3.0

Pancreatitis

Inflammation of the pancreas, or pancreatitis, is a process generally associated with the presence of stones in the gallbladder. In fact, it is one of the complications of this disease and one of the reasons why it is recommended that the patient undergoes surgery to remove the gallbladder as soon as the gallstones are diagnosed.

When one of the gallbladder stones is too large to pass through the bile duct, it blocks the flow of bile and pancreatic fluid. This begins the inflammatory process that leads to pancreatitis.

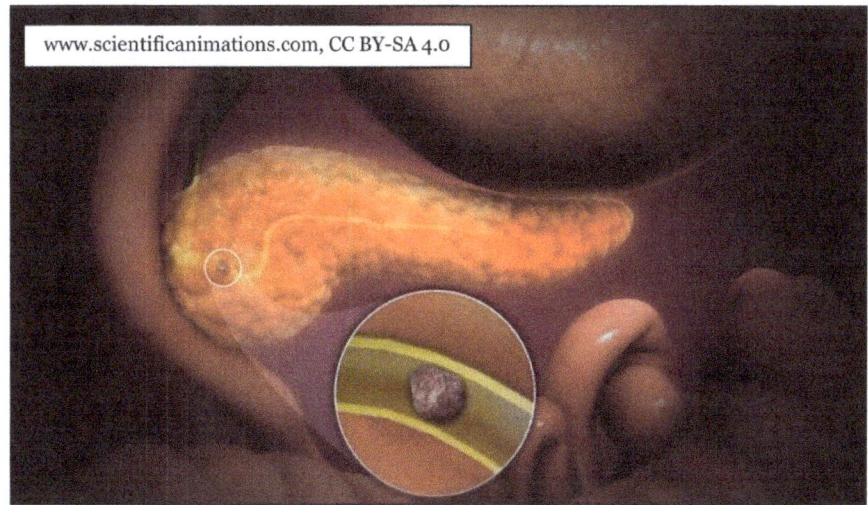

The other major cause of pancreatitis is the patient's lifestyle. Obesity, high fat intake, high triglyceride levels, above 1000mg/dL, alcohol, and smoking are all triggers for pancreatitis.

The main symptom of pancreatitis is a dull pain that wraps around the upper abdomen and involves the back. In Spanish, it is called a "bandlike pain pattern."

The definitive diagnosis is made by performing a CT scan of the abdomen that shows an enlarged pancreas and laboratory tests for pancreatic enzymes: Lipase and Amylase, which will be found to be elevated to about three times the upper limit of normal.

The problem with having a disease like pancreatitis is that its complications are serious, such as diabetes, and can even be fatal. When pancreatitis is suspected, it is important to start decreasing the intake of fats and grains to give the pancreas a rest.

The emergency service should be contacted immediately. A patient with suspected pancreatitis should be studied with the corresponding laboratory and imaging tests to corroborate the diagnosis.

In the event that the resultant pancreatitis is a gallstone obstruction, the blockage should be removed as soon as possible. This is done through a specialized study called endoscopic retrograde cholangiopancreatography (ERCP) and should not be postponed since complications include infection, sepsis, and death.

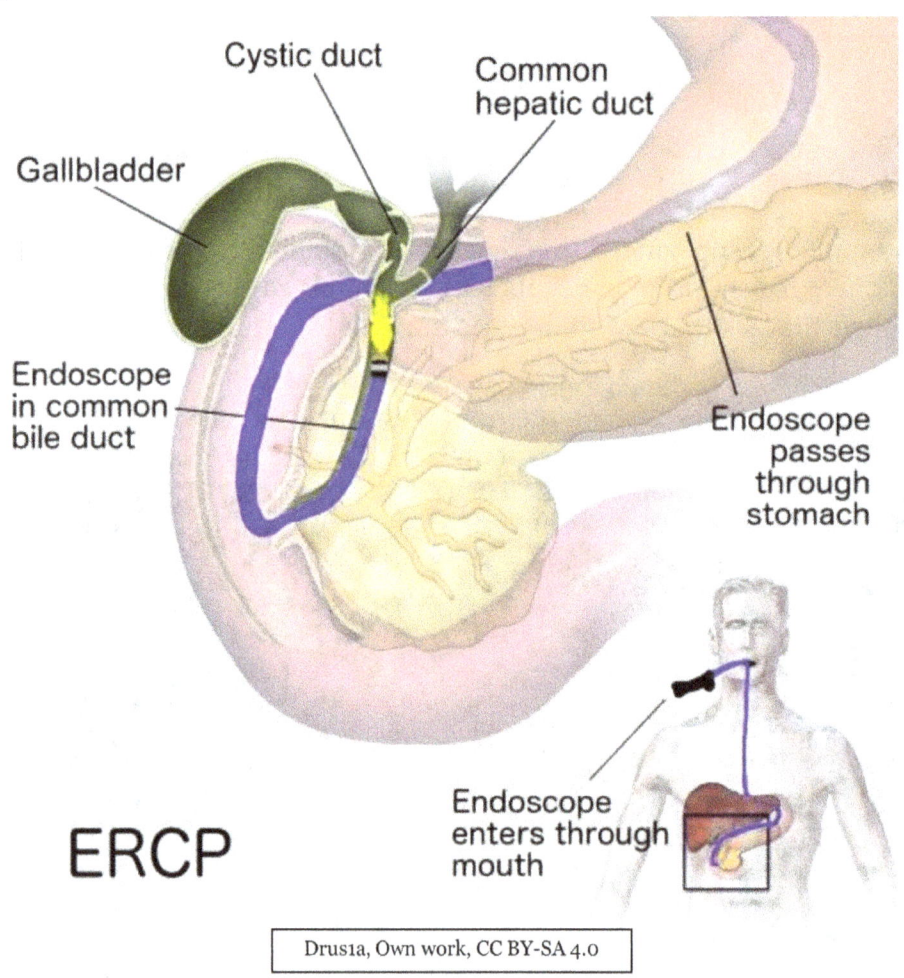

Drus1a, Own work, CC BY-SA 4.0

Pancreatitis is a medical emergency that must be treated right away. However, if this is not possible, some of the patient's signs that indicate worsening should be taken into account: fever, increased breathing rate, continuous and progressive pain, and purple on the sides and around the navel.

These signs denote necrosis and destruction of pancreatic tissue that will likely require surgery and management in the ICU.

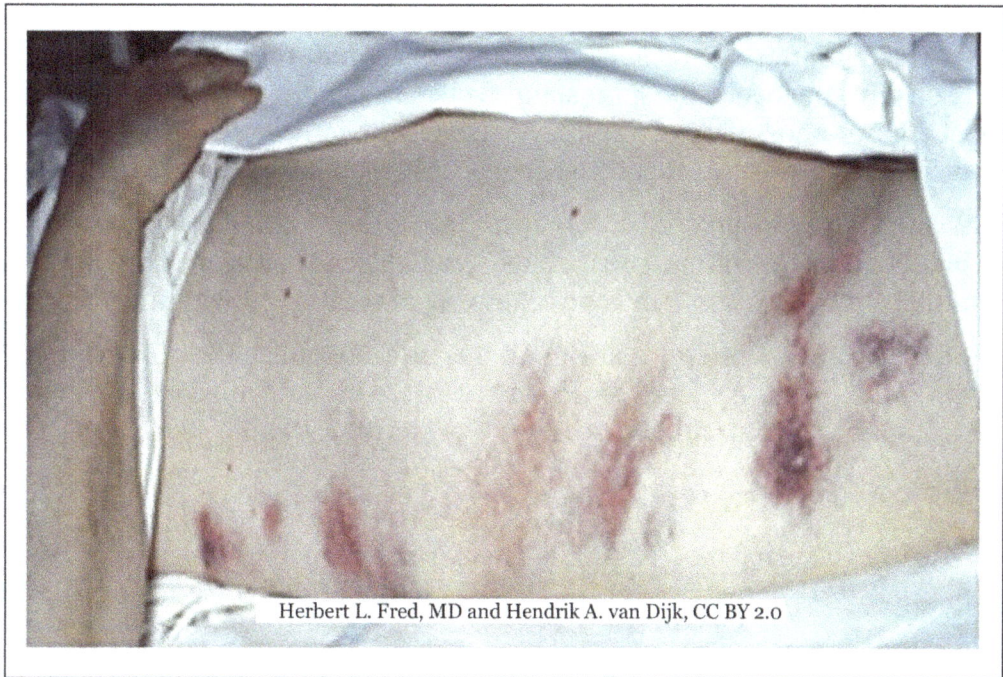

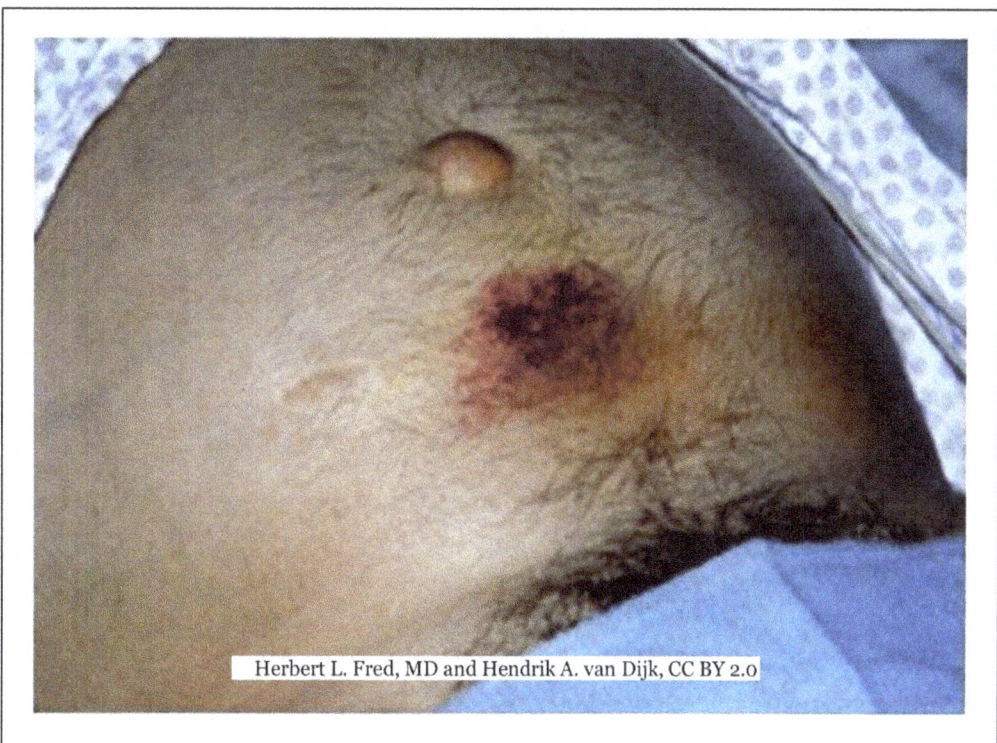

Diabetes Mellitus (DM)

Diabetes is a disease in which the patient has increased levels of glucose (blood sugar) over a long periodof time. There are two types: type 1, or juvenile, diabetes, in which the pancreatic cells do not produce insulin, and type 2 diabetes, in which the tissues lose their affinity for insulin.

The symptoms of diabetes are increased thirst (polydipsia), increased hunger (polyphagia), and increased urination. In addition, patients suffering from this condition have progressive damage to the kidneys, eyes, and sensitive nerves of the hands and feet. The patient with diabetes loses sensitivity in their hands and feet ("glove-and-stocking anesthesia"), so it is common to have wounds in these places that later become ulcers that are very difficult to heal because diabetes affects the scarring process.

Type 1 diabetes is an autoimmune disorder in which the immune system attacks the cells that produce insulin by destroying them. Its symptoms occur acutely, usually in adolescence or youth. It is also called "insulin-dependent diabetes" because there is no other way to treat it but with insulin.

Type 2 diabetes develops over time. It starts with a condition called **insulin resistance**, which is reversible with lifestyle changes. At first it can be treated with oral medication, but if the process continues to progress, insulin will eventually need to be prescribed.

a) Diagnosis

The diagnosis is made by measuring blood glucose. The normal value is 80 to 110 mg/dL. A person witha value greater than 126 mg/dL after an eight-hour fast, or greater than 200 mg/dL at any time, is considered diabetic.

The measurement can be made with a small device called a glucometer. To use it, a blood sample is taken from the fingertip and placed on a special glucose measuring tape. This tape is inserted into the glucometer to give the result.

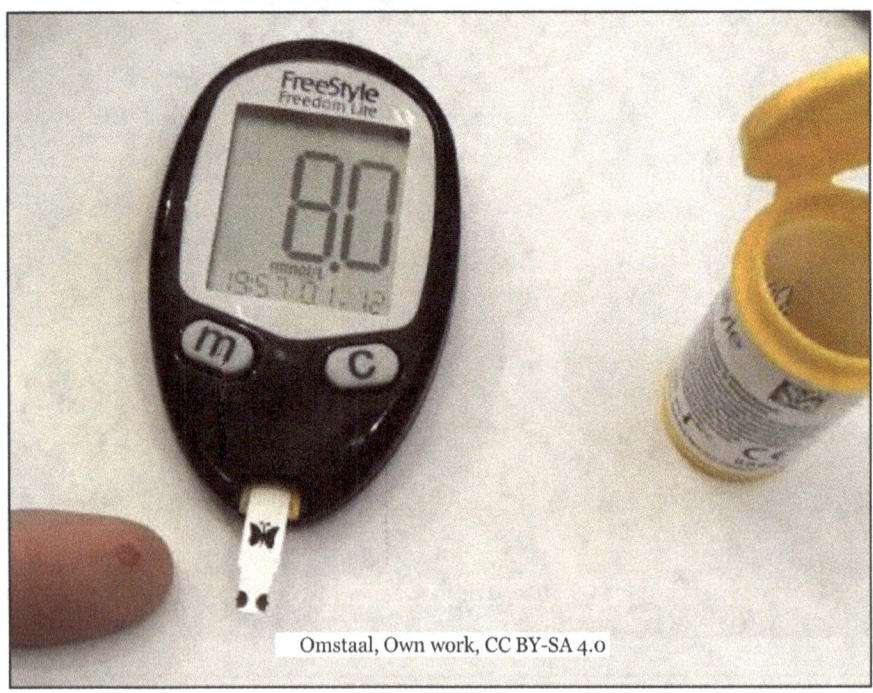

Omstaal, Own work, CC BY-SA 4.0

I always encourage my diabetic patients to have a glucometer at home as it is an excellent tool for monitoring their blood sugar values when they are not feeling well.

Symptoms such as dizziness, confusion, blurred vision, and lethargy are often manifestations of hyperglycemia. If the increase in glucose is not treated, you run the risk of suffering the complications of the disease that can trigger coma and death.

Symptoms such as increased hunger, irritability, tremors, sweating, cold, loss of consciousness, or seizures are associated with hypoglycemia. A glucose reading below 80 mg/dL is considered hypoglycemia.

This emergency can almost always be managed at home with the ingestion of a teaspoon of sugar, water with sugar, or a piece of candy. More severe cases should be hospitalized for intravenous glucose solution. Once the affected person consumes sugar, the symptoms quickly reverse, and they return to normal within minutes.

b) Treatment

There is no medicine that cures diabetes. In the case of early type 2 diabetes and insulin resistance, drugs are given that increase tissue sensitivity to this hormone. In the case of type 1 or advanced type 2 diabetes (conditions in which the cells do not produce insulin), insulin is indicated.

For patients with type 2 diabetes, there are several natural options for glycemic management. One of my aunts is diabetic, and currently, in the area where she lives far from the capital, she cannot find her treatment, so she has had to use natural medicine, which so far have proved to be quite good in combination with some dietary and physical suggestions.

BERBERINE

Berberine is an extract from the roots of several plants that has long been used as a natural medicine to treat various metabolic conditions with considerable success. Although it is not well known how it works, in the case of diabetes, its results have been studied, and there is scientific evidence that it is able to lower blood glucose levels.

It is not advisable to take it together with a hypoglycemic such as Metformin, because the effect can be very strong. That is why I recommend taking it independently, recording glycemia levels every 4 hours.

Berberine capsules 500 mg, Dosage: 1 capsule before every main meal

APPLE CIDER VINEGAR

Apple cider vinegar is one of my favorite supplements, and I take it daily for all its properties. In the case of diabetes, it improves the sensitivity of the tissues to insulin; taking it together with the usual therapy helps to manage adequate glucose levels even on an empty stomach.

I take two spoonsful mixed in on glass of water, on an empty stomach. If the taste doesn't sit well you, you can use it as a salad dressing or as a marinade for meat.

Do not take it undiluted, as it can damage the tooth enamel.

It is used to control stomach acid secretion, improve breath, and acidify skin pH. It seems to have effects on varicose veins and circulation, but they have not been completely studied.

ALPHA LIPOIC ACID

This supplement is very beneficial in the case "gloves and stocking anesthesia." Using it for three months has shown excellent results in partially recovering sensitivity.

It also has a minor effect on increasing tissue sensitivity to insulin.

Alpha Lipoic Acid (ALA) capsules 300mg, Dosage: 2 capsules daily for 3 months

Lifestyle changes have beneficial effects on the diabetic patient and can reverse insulin resistance. Losing weight and exercising daily improve the sensitivity of tissues, especially muscle, to insulin so glucose is better metabolized.

Reducing carbohydrate consumption is important since during the digestion process, carbohydrates are converted into glucose.

A colleague once taught me a technique for remembering the best foods for diabetes: "If it grows above ground, it can be consumed. If it grows under the ground, it should be eaten in moderation.

If it is white, it should be avoided. And if it walks, flies, swims, or crawls, it can be eaten."

Another important point is to get used to reading labels and not to buy the product just because it is special for diabetics.

Many times these types of foods compensate for the decrease in sugar by adding fat to maintain the flavor, so they are still harmful to your health.

2. Obesity and Metabolic Syndrome

Metabolic syndrome is a group of diseases that increase the risk of developing cardiovascular complications.

If a person has three or more of the following characteristics, metabolic syndrome is diagnosed:

- Abdominal obesity: Waist circumference greater than 40 inches in men, and 35 inches in women
- Triglyceride level of 150 mg/dL or greater
- HDL cholesterol of less than 40 mg/dL in men or less than 50 mg/dL in women
- Systolic blood pressure of 130 mm Hg or greater, or diastolic blood pressure of 85 mm Hg or greater
- Fasting glucose greater than 100 mg/dL

Each of these conditions is a risk for cardiovascular disease, but when they are part of a group, the risk increases dramatically, putting the patient's life at risk.

Metabolic syndrome can be reversed if lifestyle changes are made. If you lose weight and exercise at least 30 minutes a day, your blood pressure values will drop and your tissues will become more sensitiveto insulin, lowering your blood glucose value.

Obesity is measured by the value of the body mass index (BMI), which is calculated using the formula weight (kg) x height (meters)^2.

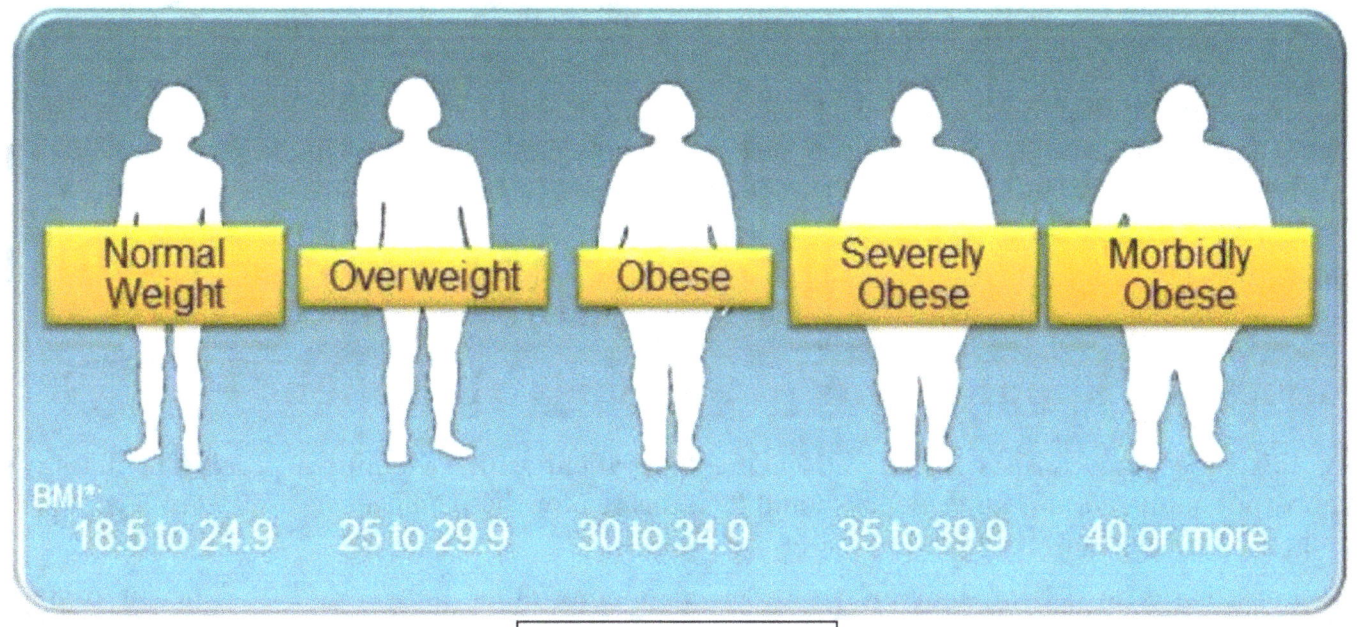

Thiruthonti, CC BY-SA 4.0

Obesity is a metabolic disease that increases the risk of hyperlipidemia and hypercholesterolemia (increased blood fats and cholesterol). In addition, it conditions the poor management of glucose as tissues tend to lose their sensitivity to insulin.

We've all known obese people who lose weight and then have a rebound effect and gain even more than they had lost. Most spend a large part of their lives this way, subjecting the body to the stress of this hormonal and systemic imbalance. These patients are the perfect candidates for obesity surgery or bariatric surgery. This procedure helps the patient to lose weight by means of the restrictive mechanism, cutting out a good part of the stomach, and the malabsorption mechanism.

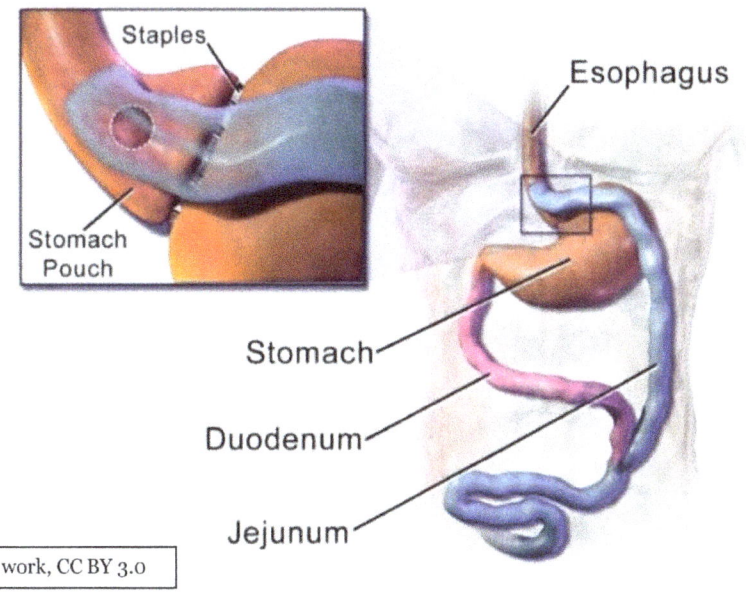

Blausen.com staff, Own work, CC BY 3.0

After bariatric surgery, patients lose approximately 50% of their weight within six months of the procedure and reach their goal weight between one and one and a half years after the surgery.

Although other bariatric techniques have been used that include only the restrictive mechanism, such as sleeve gastrectomy and gastric banding, none has shown as good of results as the gastric bypass. This is why it remains the standard for the treatment of morbid obesity.

It has been shown that after significant weight loss as well as bariatric surgery, metabolic syndrome begins to improve. Blood pressure levels improve significantly as well as glucose levels. Over time, the abdominal circumference also decreases. This eliminates all cardiovascular risk factors.

Nutritional Supplements in the Bariatric Patient

Since this procedure consists in part of leaving the patient with a definitive process of digestive malabsorption, nutritional supplements should be indicated for these deficiencies. Vitamin B complex, vitamin A, iron, and zinc are important to prevent anemia.

In the post-bariatric patient, hair loss is observed, among other things, due to deficient protein absorption, especially during the first months after surgery, when it is not easy for them to eat a complete meal.

For this reason, whey or vegetable protein supplements are indicated, according to their habits and preference, to complete the amount of daily protein needed and not to fall into malnutrition.

Currently there are specific multivitamins for post-bariatric patients that contain all the necessary vitamins at the right dose.

NERVOUS SYSTEM

The nervous system is the part of the organism that is responsible for directing the motor elements and interpreting the senses in order to function properly. Through the nervous system, we can relate to the environment around us.

It is divided into central and peripheral. The former consists of the brain and spinal cord and the latter of all the nerves and neurological cells in the body.

As it plays such an important role, diseases involving the nervous system manifest themselves with very noticeable symptoms, whether they are involuntary movements or loss of muscle strength.

When a person complains of some discomfort involving motor or sensory deficits, we must be vigilant as these may be some of the conditions affecting this system.

WHAT DAMAGES THE NERVOUS SYSTEM?

Conditions related to the nervous system can be traumatic, infectious, or degenerative. Traumatic injuries are quite frequent, and their consequences may be reversible in many cases but will depend on the type and mechanism of the injury.

Infectious diseases can be bacterial, viral, or fungal; bacterial diseases affect children more frequently. The degenerative causes are chronic diseases, such as Alzheimer's, Parkinson's disease, and multiple sclerosis, which all evolve over time.

EVALUATION OF THE NERVOUS SYSTEM: HOW DO I KNOW IF THE PATIENT IS OKAY?

The physical examination involving the nervous system is one of the most fun and logical in the field of medicine. There are no tricks or ambiguities; everything is quite clear because each nerve controls a specific part of the body, and each area if the brain has specific functions.

The examination of the nervous system begins, as always, with questioning. This is followed by a physical examination, which in this case involves muscle-tendon reflexes, sensitivity, and muscle strength.

By simply talking to the person, we are already assessing the brain areas and their temporal and spatial orientation. Questions such as "What day is it?", "What year is it?", or "What is your full name?" tell us if the patient has any level of amnesia or confusion.

Muscle strength is assessed by asking the patient to squeeze your hands simultaneously with full force. Lower limb strength is also tested with the patient sitting up and pushing up while you try to lower the leg.

In medicine, when we examine paired organs, it's all about comparison.

The sensitivity of the skin is examined with a sharp element and a soft one (it can be a needle and a cotton ball); that way we can know if the person has lost sensitivity and to what degree.

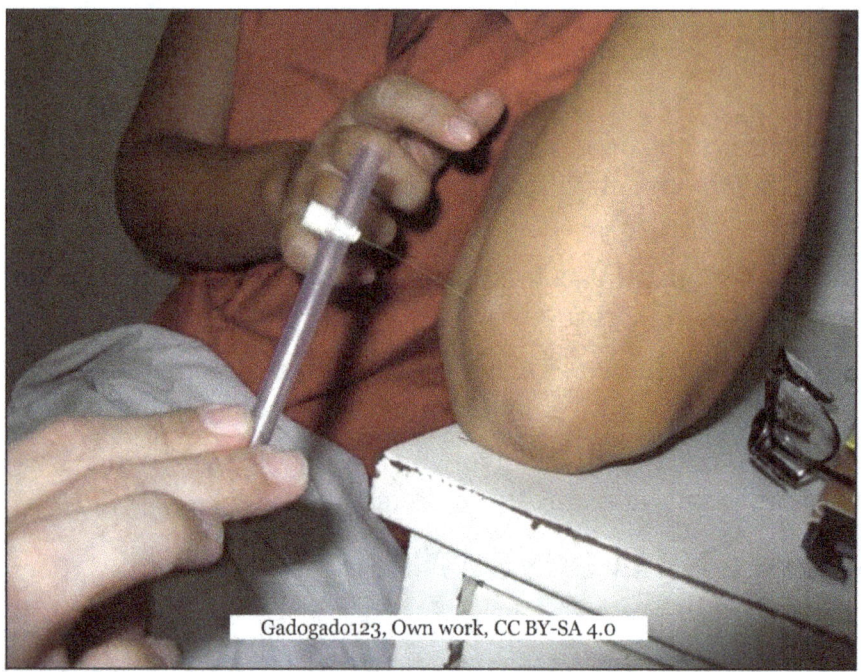

Gadogado123, Own work, CC BY-SA 4.0

There are conditions in which the cotton ball cannot be felt but the needle stick can be felt. These changes have different interpretations. You have to be meticulous.

There are professional tools, such as the *neurological hammer*, that come with some items to evaluate sensitivity.

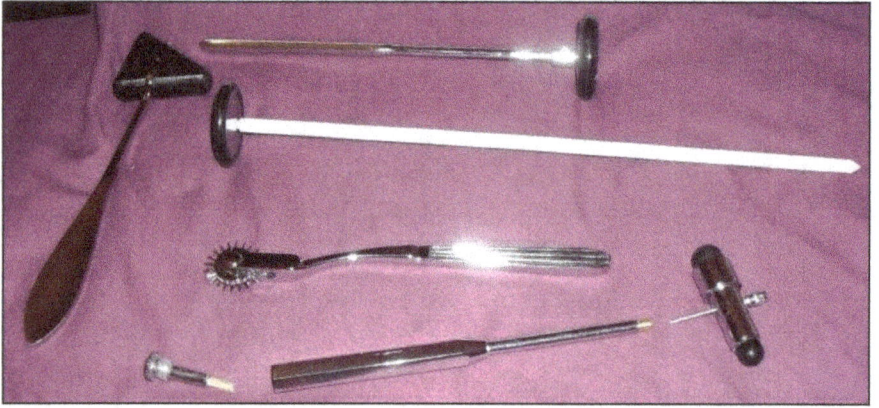

Ali Raheem, Own work, CC BY-SA 3.0

With the hammer, which is actually a strong rubber mallet, you can evaluate the skin muscle reflexes. The easiest one is the knee, or patellar, reflex, and it helps us to see the proper functioning of the communication between the brain and the muscles.

With the patient seated, take his or her leg behind the knee and strike the ligament between the knee and the leg with the hammer. This forces the person you are examining to kick involuntarily.

My idea is not to teach you a professional neurological exam but to show you the basics so that you can make a diagnostic approach and understand how serious the situation is that you are facing.

1. Stroke

A stroke is a medical emergency that requires immediate attention. Sometimes it brings serious complications, and sometimes it can be resolved without major problems.

Not all strokes lead to death or paralysis. Even when the patient is left with some consequences, a high percentage can improve completely with the help of physical or verbal therapy.

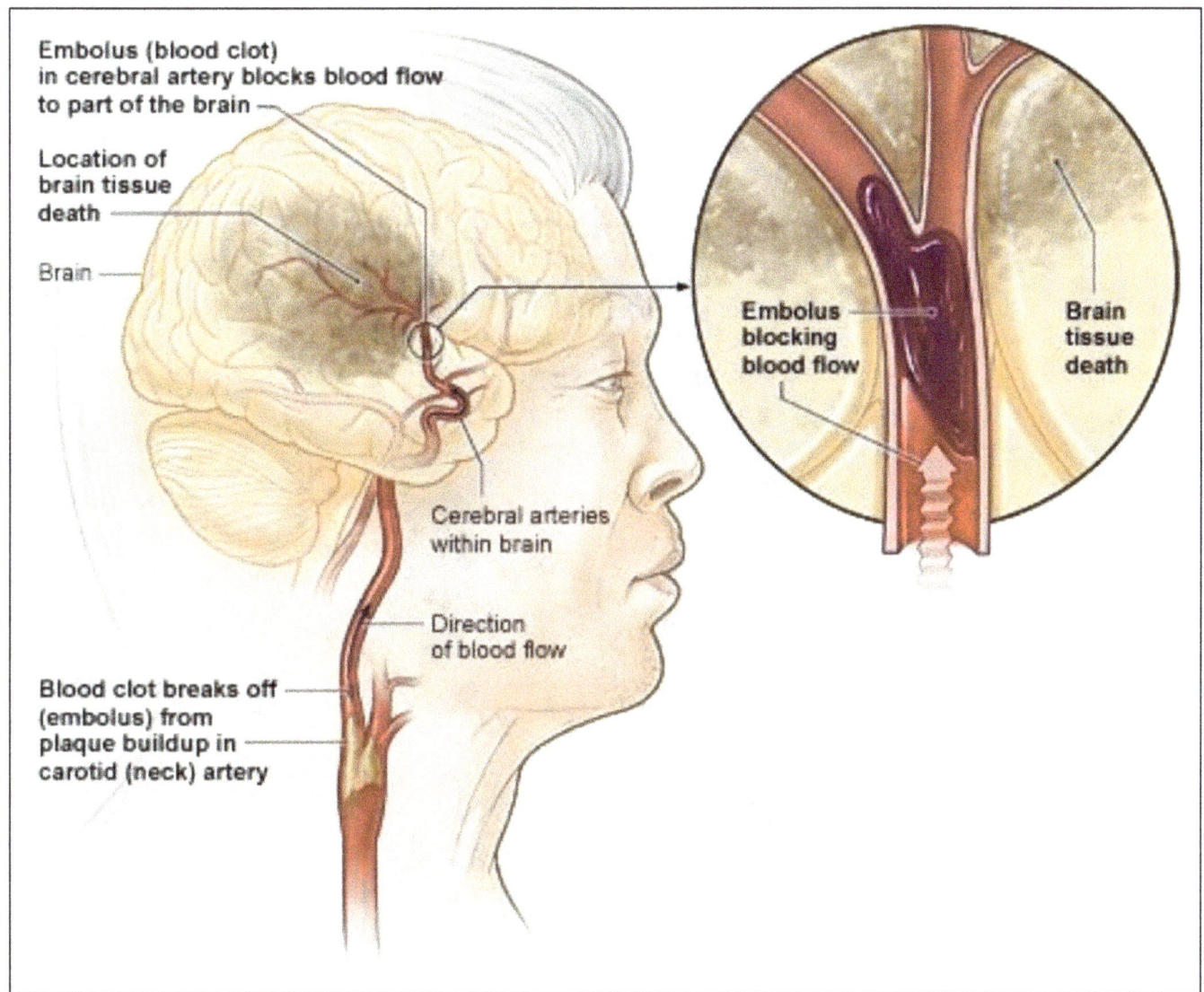

Ischemic strokes occur because a blockage in the artery prevents blood from flowing normally to the brain.

This can be due to local damage, fatty plaques (atherosclerosis) inside the artery, or a clot that forms in the heart and travels through the larger arteries but gets trapped in the smaller ones.

Symptoms

Ischemic stroke causes a heart attack in an area of the brain. This means that the blood supply is stopped because of a blockage in an artery that reaches a specific area of the brain.

The symptoms will depend on the area affected, but there are three symptoms that are common to all ischemic strokes. The best way to learn the symptoms to identify an ischemic stroke is through the mnemonic **FAST**. This acronym stands for:

- **F**ace drooping
- **A**rm weakness
- **S**peech difficulty
- **T**ime to call 911

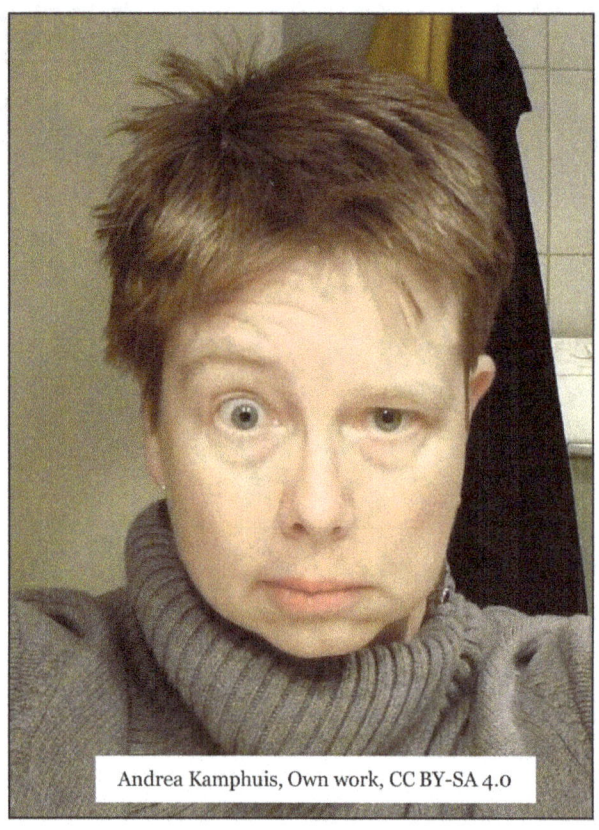

Andrea Kamphuis, Own work, CC BY-SA 4.0

In the photo above, you can see the asymmetry in the patient's facial expression. On one side, she can open her eye wide and expression lines can be seen, while on the other side, the mouth is fallen, the eye is halfway closed, and her forehead is not wrinkled.

No matter what area of the brain is affected, these symptoms will always be present and must be recognized.

IF A STROKE IS SUSPECTED, IT IS ABSOLUTELY NECESSARY TO CALL 911.

2. Seizures

Seizures are sudden, involuntary movements that occur because of a problem in the brain's electrical activity. The movements are most clearly seen in the arms, hands, and in the face. The lips tend to make a movement that resembles suction. The expressionless face and dilated pupils are also obvious signs that the person is having a seizure.

Working as a general practitioner, I was able to attend to several seizure episodes in non-epileptic patients, which was a relatively frequent reason for consultation. A seizure can be triggered by drug interactions, especially psychotropic drugs such as Tramadol, a fever over 100°, head trauma, and strokes. Some people suffer from epilepsy, which is a condition characterized by periodic seizures. These patients are usually diagnosed at an early age and maintain lifelong treatment.

How Do I Know Someone Is Having a Seizure and What Should I Do?

Recognizing a seizure is easy. It is an unconscious patient with repetitive, jerky movements who expels large amounts of saliva from the mouth, like foam. These movements make the muscles very tight and can cause the person to hit their head and bite their tongue, causing injury.

During a seizure, you should try to stay calm. Before you call for emergency services, it is important to treat the patient so that he does not hurt himself.

A seizure can take less than a minute. During that time, it is necessary to assist the patient. The 911 call should be made, but it is essential to attend to the urgent situation.

Place the patient in a horizontal position, and put the head to the side to prevent choking on saliva or the tongue. If the seizure is starting, you can tuck a tissue between the teeth to prevent tongue damage.

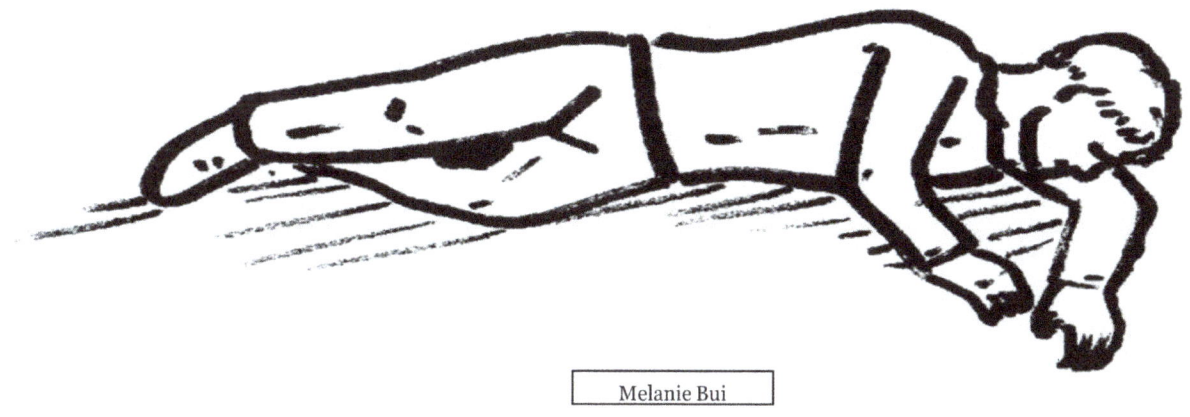
Melanie Bui

Check for details such as sphincter relaxation, meaning involuntary urination or evacuation, and keep track of the time the seizure lasts. This will be important information for the emergency team.

After the seizure, the patient may be very confused, with amnesia of the last minutes before the episode, and sleepy. Try to calm them down and explain what happened while waiting for professional help.

IMMUNE SYSTEM

The immune system is a defense structure that acts to protect the host. The human immune system is complex and consists of two parts, one innate and primitive, which is with us from birth, and another that is learned by specialized cells for that purpose.

The skin is our main barrier against the adverse elements of the environment. It is the largest and most visible organ of the immune system. We develop protection against allergens, bacteria, viruses, and other microorganisms over time.

A newborn baby has been exposed to almost nothing, so it only possesses the primitive immunity and some cells of the mother's immune system.

This is why the mother's care during pregnancy is always encouraged, including a good diet and prenatal vitamins, since these cells are the ones that will help the newborn during the first weeks, along with the breastmilk.

The human being has several organs that are specifically responsible for immunity through the creation of antibodies against the pathogens we face. That's actually how vaccines work in the body.

For example, a 20-year-old person will have already had several diseases, such as flu and maybe chicken pox. However, if he is faced with a new pathogen that his system does not recognize, he will have a mild immune response.

But that pathogen within the body is studied by specific cells with cellular memory. These memory cells, which already know the pathogen, are cloned into some of the organs of the immune system, and that patient is protected from further infection by that organism.

Another example is when young children leave the house to start school or daycare. The first few days, dealing with other children and a different environment from home will lead you to get small infectionsin a row, over a period of time.

After a couple of months that same child can be with his peers without any health problems.

1. What Can Disturb My Immune System?

In addition to the diseases of immunity, there are everyday situations that weaken our immune systems. Stress, which has been called the "epidemic of cities," tops that list. I am among those who live in the midst of work and housework, without much time for leisure. While keeping busy is important for many of us in our professional development, it's not the best for the body. Like fatigue, when the body needs a break, it simply puts different mechanisms to work to get you to stop for a while.

Poor nutrition is a major trigger of disease because of low defenses. Food is fundamental in the process of cell formation. Without adequate nutrition, the little the body can salvage as fuel is directed to the vital organs, leaving the rest neglected. Thus, malnutrition can lead to anemia, and low defenses are the logical consequence.

Malnutrition brings many associated problems, some of which are infection with opportunistic pathogens. These types of microorganisms are those that under normal conditions rarely enter the body.

However, they take advantage of any situation of diminishing protective barriers to make their triumphant entry. Some types of fungi, tuberculosis, and some skin infections, among others, are some of these infections.

2. How Do I Strengthen My Immune System?

Simple habit changes, such as daily exercise, will keep your immune system at acceptable levels. If you add to that a proper diet consisting of proteins, whether animal or vegetable; healthy fats; and vegetables, you can be sure that you will stay healthy.

However, there are some foods that help us strengthen and maintain our defenses at 100% of their potential. If we cannot leave the house and we cannot exercise as we are used to, it is necessary to keep our defenses at the highest possible level.

One of my favorite recipes is **golden milk**. This is an Indian drink that goes back thousands of years. It has been used as an anti-inflammatory, digestive aid, and relaxing and restorative sleep aid. I prepare it by mixing in a cup of milk (I use almonds), two tablespoons of turmeric, one tablespoon of cinnamon, a teaspoon of freshly ground black pepper, and ginger.

Green tea is another of my favorite drinks. It's a top-notch antioxidant as well as a diuretic. It increases the rate of metabolism and is an aid to the oxidation of body fat. I do not recommend taking it after 5:00 p.m. as in some people it has an excitatory effect on the central nervous system.

Vitamin C is absolutely necessary in the defense against daily pathogens and even more so against new ones. Do not exceed the daily vitamin C consumption however.

The recommended daily amount of vitamin C is 90 milligrams for adult men and 75 milligrams for adult women. Many, many foods contain it, and there are also many supplements.

We all know that citrus fruits contain vitamin C; however, few know that broccoli, spinach, and brussels sprouts are among the most complete foods in terms of the supply of this specific vitamin.

In my country, there is no shortage of the famous **chicken foot soup** when it comes to raising the defenses and fighting any kind of ailment. This extra-collagenous preparation has many benefits at an immunological level and, above all, at a bone level. If you are adventurous, dare to give it a try.

As you have realized throughout this book, **garlic** is one of the foods with the most properties, so of course, it improves the immune system. Whether you start adding it to your food, drink it as a tea, or take it in capsules if you don't like the taste, it will give you all the benefits this food provides.

Garlic capsules 500 mg, Dosage: 2 daily

Acai is a fruit I was familiar with in the Amazon. They use it for many purposes, from food to ornamentals. I had seen this fruit many times growing on the palms one finds on the beach. However, I had never paid attention to it, so I didn't even know it was edible. They say this fruit strengthens and restores your defenses if you've been in the rain or in the river for a long time. Its consumption is also indicated in the elderly and in people with muscle or joint pain. It can be eaten fresh with the skin, andit tastes great. A few years ago, it became very popular in the world of fitness as it is considered a superfood that provides excellent nutritional and health benefits. From that moment on, this fruit has been named much more in preparations such as smoothies and fruit bowls. Where fresh fruit is not available, there are liquid, capsule, and powder supplements that will also give you the benefits of the fruit.

Acai capsules 300 mg, Dosage: 2 daily

Finally, I must mention that rest is absolutely necessary to maintain good health, not only immunological but general health. Some techniques that I recommend are establishing the time of sleep and trying to achieve a routine in which you sleep at the same hour every night and/or do activities before you go to sleep that send your body the message that it is getting close to the time of rest. Try to stick to it as much as possible, and you will see very positive improvement.

A FEW RECIPES PUT TOGETHER FOR YOU

1. A Natural DIY Antibiotic Salve Recipe to Keep Around

There are several OTC antiseptic ointments to choose from at the local market, which are normally applied directly to the wound. They are meant to prevent infection from developing. While these options often work and the products have some helpful ingredients, they also have some unnecessary ingredients, so they can be mass-produced.

Fortunately, there is an alternative for those of you who choose to live a more natural life, without the unnecessary added ingredients to everyday products. This isn't about saving money, because to be honest, the ingredients are not necessarily inexpensive for the initial purchase.

On the other hand, they will last a very long time and make several batches of antiseptic. Or, you can share by making this for family and friends who also want to benefit from a purer approach to healing.

Making the Ointment

The recipe we are sharing is packed with anti-germ properties, which will aid in keeping a minor wound from becoming infected. It will also help in reducing any possible scarring.

The ingredients are well-known for their healing tendencies, as well as their effectiveness in fighting off infections. So, combining them into a natural homemade ointment to have on hand just makes sense.

Here is the list of ingredients you will need:

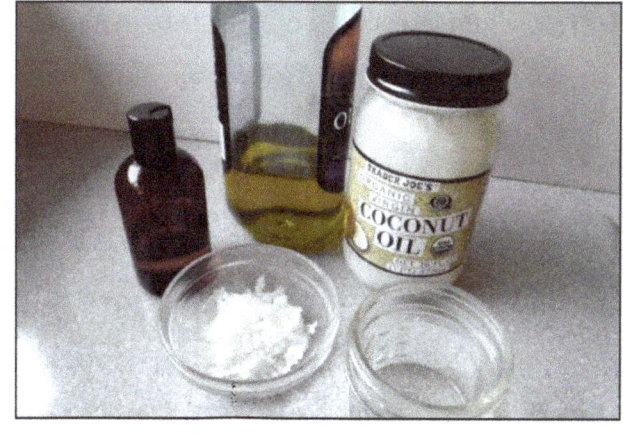

- 5 oz. beeswax (pellets melt quicker)
- 1 cup almond oil (could replace this with olive or coconut oil)
- 0.5 tsp. tea tree oil
- 25 drops vitamin E oil
- 20 drops of lavender essential oil
- 10 drops of lemon essential oil.

But, before we discuss the steps in making this ointment, it's good to know why each of these ingredients is important:

- *Lavender Essential Oil* not only soothes, but also works as a pain reliever, antibiotic, anti-viral, anti-fungal, and antibacterial.
- *Tea Tree Oil* is known for its anti-fungal, anti-viral, antibiotic, and anti-bacterial properties.

- *Lemon Essential Oil* acts as an antibiotic, anti-viral, anti-fungal, and anti-bacterial.
- *Vitamin E Oil* aids in healing the skin and reducing any scarring that might occur from a minor injury.
- *Almond Oil* has helped a few people heal breakouts of various skin conditions.

Now that you know how each ingredient contributes to making this ointment work, here are the easy directions to putting them all together in creating a healthy and useful antiseptic ointment.

Step 1: In a small pot, melt the beeswax and almond oil on a very low heat setting.

Step 2: Once that has melted, take the pot off the heat source.

Step 3: Add the tea tree oil, vitamin E oil, lavender oil, and lemon oil, stirring with a wooden spoon.

Step 4: After the mixture is blended, pour it into a small and sterilized container, and let it cool.

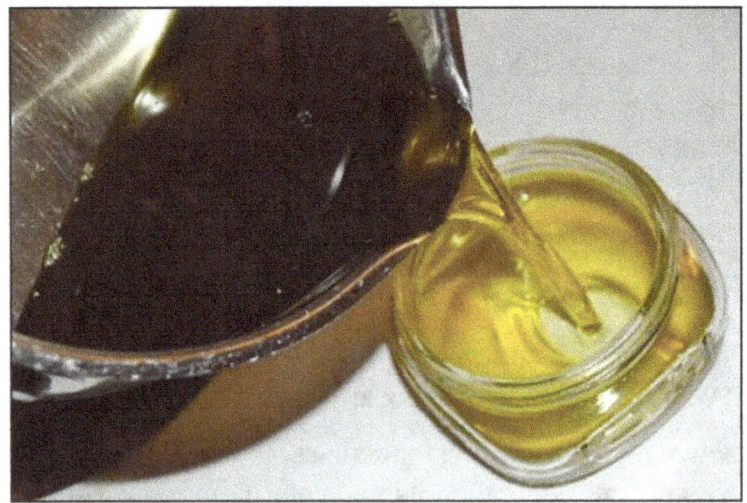

Step 5: When it's cooled down, store in a cool and dark place.

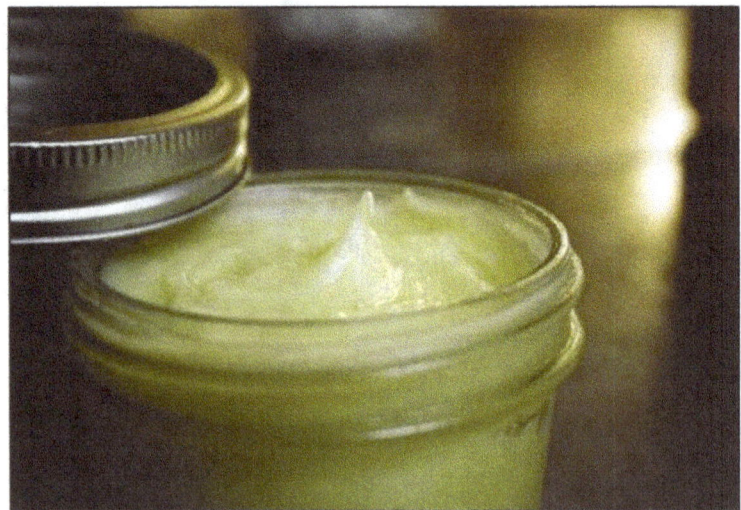

That is all there is to it – a very simple way to make an ointment for minor wounds. If you experience a minor cut, scratch, or abrasion, dab a little bit of this ointment on the wound a couple of times a day until it is healed. This ointment has a shelf life of about five years. On a side note, for those who do not like the smell of lemon or lavender, you can substitute either one, or both. Lavender can be replaced with chamomile essential oil, and lemon can be replaced with fir essential oil.

2. A Simple "At-Home" Protocol for the Flu and Other Respiratory Issues

Viruses are a part of life that humans have had to live with for centuries. Many viruses can affect us year-round, but during the winter months, flu and other respiratory viruses seem to get worse and cause more issues. There are many reasons for this.

First, the lack of sunlight causes a deficiency in vitamin D. Vitamin D is necessary to keep our immune systems strong. Make sure that you are taking a vitamin D supplement during the darker months. In addition to less sunlight, our bodies become bogged down by unhealthy eating during all those holidays and lack of exercise since many of us become cooped up indoors due to cooler temperatures. Try to remain active and eat healthy, whole foods as much as possible.

If and when you do happen to come down with a respiratory virus, you can take steps to help your body heal and recover quickly. You can even do this in the comfort of your own home! The remedies below have been used to strengthen the immune system and body for centuries. In addition, many of the ingredients just might already be in your pantry.

1. Old-Fashioned Fire Cider

Nobody is completely sure where the term "fire cider" came from, but herbalists around the globe have been preparing this special concoction for many years to fight various viruses. Fire cider recipes differ between herbalists and countries, but many require the use of spicy plants that stimulate the immune system and speed up recovery.

<u>Fire Cider Recipe</u>

For this recipe, you will need:

- Glass jar
- Jar rim lid
- Cheesecloth
- Raw, unfiltered apple cider vinegar
- Three to four jalapenos
- Two to three cayenne peppers
- Chopped onion
- A few sprigs of thyme

#1. Place all the chopped plant ingredients in a glass jar.
#2. Completely cover the plant material in apple cider vinegar.
#3. Place cheesecloth over the top and then secure it on with the jar rim lid.
#4. Let this sit in a cool, dark place for four weeks before straining it out. Bottle the liquid and take aone ounce shot at the onset of a virus and every few hours as needed for stimulating the immune system.

2. Killing a Cough

If you just can't seem to shake a cough, give this recipe a try. This recipe is made from common household items and can be whipped up fast if you need relief. If a cough is keeping you up at night, follow the steps below:

Quick Cough Relief Syrup For

this recipe, you will need:

- Small glass
- Apple cider vinegar
- Raw honey or molasses

#1. Add one half teaspoon of apple cider vinegar to the glass.
#2. Add one teaspoon of raw honey or molasses to the glass.
#3. Add one fourth teaspoon of ground ginger to the glass. **#4.**
Add one fourth teaspoon of ground cinnamon to the glass.**#5.**
Squeeze the juice of a half a lemon into the glass.
#6. Stir everything together well.
#7. Drink this mixture, but gargle it a little in the back of your throat as you swallow it. This will helpto coat and soothe the throat and prevent coughing fits.

3. Homemade Onion Cough Syrup

Onion and honey are two wonderful ingredients from nature. Both of these have strong anti-inflammatory properties and are great as a home remedy for fighting both colds and the flu. Besides having strong anti-inflammatory properties, honey and onion are also good for your immune system. So, at the first sign of flu, grab this onion syrup and suppress those viruses that are trying to make you ill. Onions are antimicrobial, anti-inflammatory, and immune stimulating.

For this recipe, you will need:

- Glass Jar with non-metal lid (as the honey has an acidic pH and reacts with metallic surfaces)
- Onion to fit in the container
- Raw Honey (preferably local).

#1. Layer honey and fresh cut onion slices in a jar.

#2. Make sure the onion slices are fully covered in honey.

#3. Seal the jar tightly, and let it sit at room temperature for 1 to 2 days.

#4. If you want to use it sooner, you can start using it within 12 hours.

#5. Ready to use! Simply eat a spoonful of this syrup as needed to soothe your cough. Store in the refrigerator.

Note: You can strain out the onions once the syrup is done, but it is not necessary.

4. Medicinal Pickled Garlic

Garlic is a wonderful ingredient from nature. It has strong anti-inflammatory properties and it is great as a home remedy for fighting both colds and the flu. Besides having strong anti-inflammatory properties, garlic is also good for the immune system. So, at the first sign of flu, grab this pickled garlic, or even garlic clove, and suppress those viruses that are trying to make you ill. Garlic is filled with allicin, a compound known to have anti-microbial properties. Apple cider vinegar contains prebiotic pectin, an essential for good digestion, which helps foster the growth of probiotics in the gut. Raw honey is also a prebiotic food that may promote healthy gut flora.

How to Prepare Medicinal Pickled Garlic

For this recipe, you will need:

- Peeled garlic cloves
- 1 cup of Apple Cider Vinegar (Raw, organic apple cider vinegar is ideal)
- 1 cup of Raw Local Honey.

#1. Fill a jar with the cloves (Leave 1-inch space from the top of the jar) and pour apple cider vinegar until they are completely covered.

#2. You may prefer to experiment by adding a little honey to customize the flavor.

#3. Put the lid on and close it. Leave the jar at room temperature for 1 to 2 weeks, then move it to a cellar or other cold, dark storage.

#4. You may need to "burp" the lids a few times over the first couple of days to release any built-up pressure in the jars.

You can wait at least 2 to 3 weeks before eating, but you can try it in order to discover your preferred taste. You can eat a clove of the garlic whenever you wish. In case of a cold or flu you can eat about 3-5 cloves a day.

5. What Happens If You Put Garlic in Honey?

Garlic and honey are two wonderful ingredients from nature. Both of these have strong anti-inflammatory properties and are great as a home remedy for fighting both colds and the flu. Besides having strong anti-inflammatory properties, honey and garlic are also good for your immune system. So, at the first sign of flu, grab this garlic-infused honey, or even garlic clove, and suppress those viruses that are trying to make you ill. Garlic is filled with allicin, a compound known to have anti-microbial properties.

Fermented Honey Garlic Recipe

For this recipe, you will need 1 cup garlic cloves (peeled) and 1 ½ cups honey (I used acacia).

#1. Peel the garlic and place it into a clean jar.

#2. Drizzle the honey over the garlic. You can pour the honey directly over the garlic or drizzle in by using the wooden honey spoon. Do not use a metal spoon as the honey has an acidic pH and reacts with metallic surfaces.

#3. Once the garlic is covered with the honey, place a lid on the jar.

#4. Make sure the cloves are covered in honey. You can flip the closed jar upside down and place it in a dark place.

Within a few days, the fermentation will begin. Bubbles will appear. This is the first sign your garlic is ready to consume. (Of course, you can wait a few days more or even weeks, until the honey is thinned down and garlic drops to the bottom of the jar).

6. The Surprisingly Soothing Power of Eggs

Have you ever sipped on a glass of eggnog and thought "This will surely soothe my sore throat!"? Yeah, me neither.

Apparently, we should think again.

This concoction of egg yolk, honey, and milk, served while still warm, can be a real saver.

Egg and Honey Drink Recipe

#1. Heat 2 cups of whole milk in a medium saucepan over medium heat, whisking constantly.

#2. Separate 1 egg, pour the yolk into a bowl and gently beat it with 2 teaspoons honey.

#3. Put an ounce or so of hot milk into the egg mixture and whisk well. This tempers the yolk and prevents it from scrambling in the pot. Pour the egg mixture into the pot and whisk for about 30 seconds, until frothy.

#4. Pour the final results into a cup and sprinkle some cinnamon if you want. Drink it while it is still warm. Your throat will thank you for it.

7. Homemade Onion and Walnuts Syrup

Onion contains allicin, a compound that's a strong, natural antibiotic. It can also reduce inflammation and loosen phlegm, making cough more productive. Meanwhile, the outer skins of onion provide an excellent source of vitamins A, C, E, and numerous antioxidants. The skins of onions are also a rich source of flavonoids, particularly quercetin, a potent antioxidant and anti-inflammatory. Walnuts are also very healthy and nutritious. They contain a large amount of minerals, vitamins, antioxidants and Omega 3.

This onion and walnuts syrup is simple, cheap, easy to do and it can be consumed to strengthen the immune system and help alleviate cough symptoms and sore throat.

For this recipe, you will need:

- 5 yellow onions;
- 3 whole walnuts;
- 2 cups of water (16.6 oz.).

#1. Wash the onions and cut them in four.

#2. Wash the nuts and crush them gently, so they remain almost whole.

#3. Put the onions and nuts in a pot with 2 cups of water and slowly bring them to a boil. Boil them for 30 minutes until the water lowers to half and syrup gets thicker.

#4. Strain out the onions and nuts and pour the syrup into a jar. If you want, you can also add honey, when the syrup is not warm anymore. You can keep it in a refrigerator and use it in the next 7 days. You can drink 3-4 tablespoons per day.

3. How to Make Calcium Pills from Eggshells

Many of us were brought up to eat eggs reasonably carefully, making sure that we didn't accidentally eat a piece of shell. In fact, as long as it's small enough to go down safely, it probably would do more good than harm! Eggshells are a brilliant source of calcium. Consisting of 95% calcium carbonate, the composition of essential minerals can be enormously beneficial to our bones and teeth.

Many chicken owners grind up the shells and feed them back to their chooks. If that's what you do, then hold back a few to supplement your own diet! If you buy your eggs, then for the purpose of making these supplements, search out organic, free-range eggs if possible.

How to Take it, How to Make it

The supplement couldn't be easier to make. You're basically aiming to grind the clean eggshells into a very fine powder, so that it can be taken easily.

We generally need around 1000 – 1500 mg. of Calcium every day (1 tsp. of eggshell powder equals around 1000 mg.). While it's possible to get some of that from a balanced diet, taking a supplement can sometimes be necessary.

Calcium carbonate is more bioavailable when taken in doses of no more 500 mg. at one time, so you could aim for two or three doses throughout the day, unless you've been guided by a medical professional to aim for anything more or less than a standard dose.

Another way of storing eggshell powder is to make up your own batch of supplements, by filling empty capsules (gelatin and vegetable cellulose types are widely available online) using a paper funnel and storing in a clean, dry jar.

You'll need:

- Eggshells – as many as you can use/have
- An electric or manual coffee/spice grinder, or pestle and mortar
- Clean, dry jar with lid
- Empty supplement capsules (optional).

Method:

1. Use your eggs as usual, but retain the shells. Wash them in hot water, removing any dirt. Don't take out the membrane inside – it's rich in minerals.

2. Boil the shells for five minutes and leave to dry. You can place them in an oven set to a low heat for 15 minutes, if you want to speed things up.

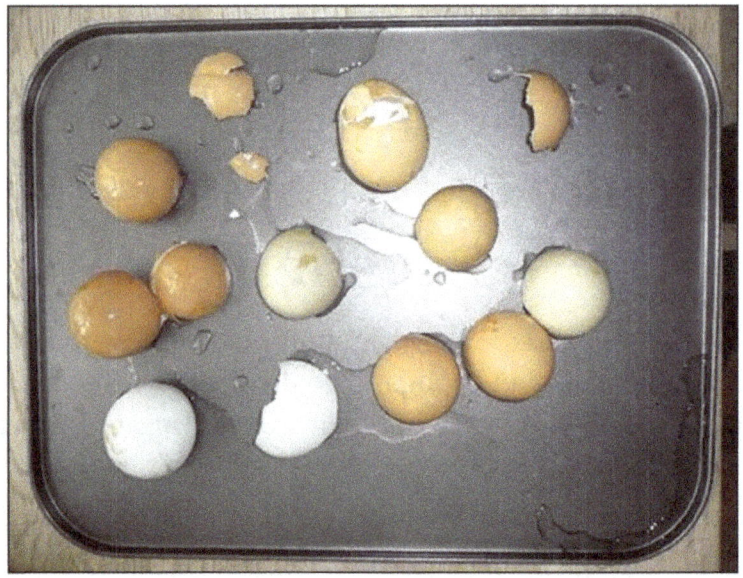

3. Once completely dry, place in your pestle and mortar or grinder and grind/pound to a very fine powder.

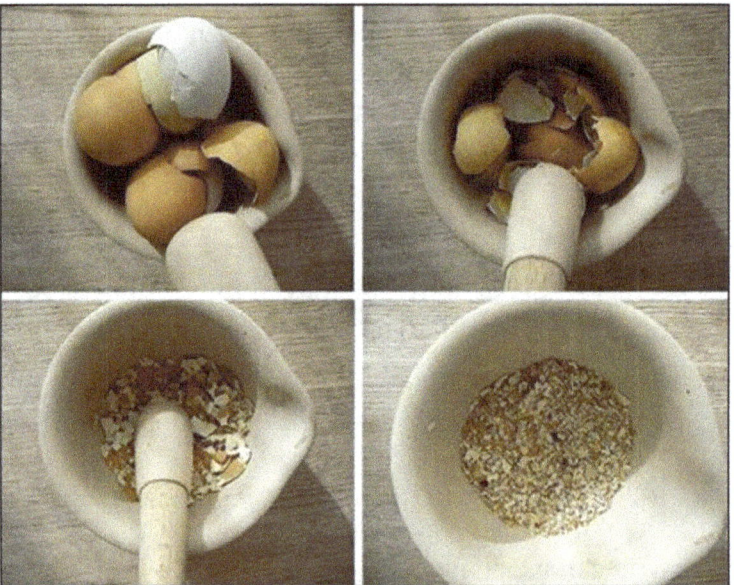

4. Sieve to remove any remaining large particles and place into a clean, dry jar with a lid.

5. If you want to fill empty capsules, then secure one half of each of the capsules using non-toxic putty or dough as a base.

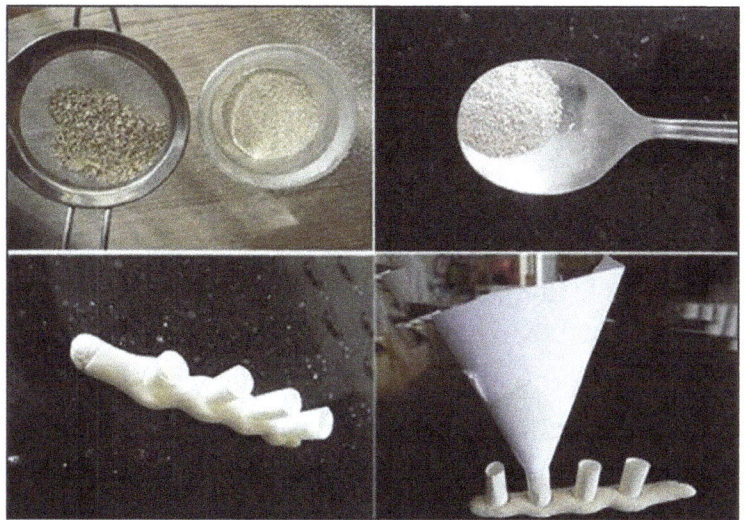

6. Now make a paper cornet and fill the capsules, then store them in a clean, dry jar.

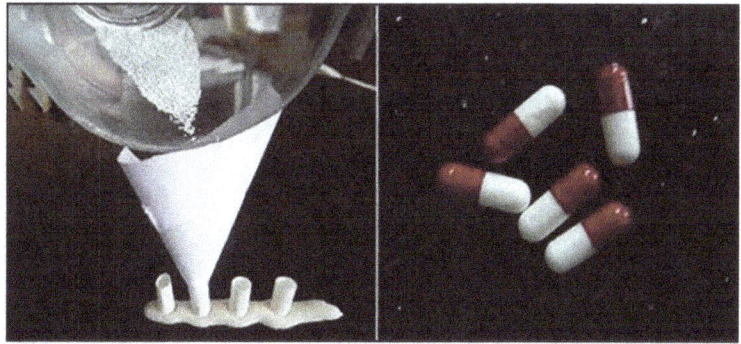

Uses and Calcium Supplement Shelf Life

It's believed that the calcium carbonate in the eggshell powder becomes more bioavailable when added to certain other foods and liquids. Vinegar, lemon juice and live yoghurt are all good for that. Many people sprinkle the powder on cereal – particularly granola or muesli – or mix it into a fruit smoothie-type drink.

In fact, the latter option is a particularly good one. If you add a banana to a homemade smoothie, the magnesium it contains helps with bioavailability and calcium absorption.

Eggshell powder has other uses too – some add it to toothpaste or mix it with a little coconut oil for a natural exfoliator.

Kept dry and out of direct sunlight, the calcium powder should last for 2 months, possibly more. If you unscrew the jar and it smells bad, then start again – it's possible that some moisture got in there.

PLANTS WITH MEDICINAL PROPERTIES

There are circumstances, such as the current worldwide pandemic, in which conventional pharmaceuticals may not be available due to a higher demand, less manpower available to produce, etc. In these times, it is practically invaluable to have information at your fingertips you can use to pinpoint the right treatment for various issues, even if you do not have access to a certain medication.

As an alternative to some pharmaceuticals, it is entirely possible to use medicinal plants in these situations. When prepared and used properly, medicinal plants can act like antibiotics, painkillers, antivirals, and anti-inflammatory drugs.

Below, you will learn what plants to use in place of various pharmaceuticals, should you ever find yourself in a situation where you don't have access to what you need.

1. Painkillers

Below is a list of plants that act as painkillers, similar to over-the-counter pain relievers. However, the plants below do not have the liver and kidney-harming side effects that many over-the-counter painkillers possess.

1. **Wild Lettuce, *Lactuca canadensis*, *L. virosa* and *L. serriola***

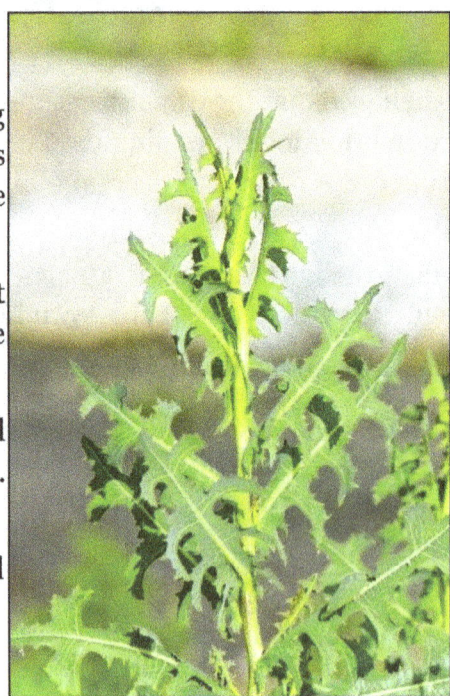

Through the ages, wild lettuce has been utilized for its painkilling abilities. It is said by some to have an "opiate-like" effect on pain. It is the white ooze inside the plant that is responsible for these attributes.

One of the best ways to prepare this very common "weed" is to boil it down into a decoction. Harvest the aerial parts of this plant and use the stem and leaves in your decoction.

Take one cup of finely chopped fresh leaves and stems (anything full of the milky substance) and add it to a pot with two cups of water. Let this boil down until only one cup of water is left.

Stir continually to avoid scorching. Strain out the plant material when it has cooled a bit and bottle this decoction.

Drink one ounce every four hours as needed for pain.

2. Valerian Root, *Valeriana officinalis*

Valerian root acts as a Central Nervous System depressant, helping to relax the body and keep nerves calm. As a result, valerian root has been proven successful at treating nerve-related pain.

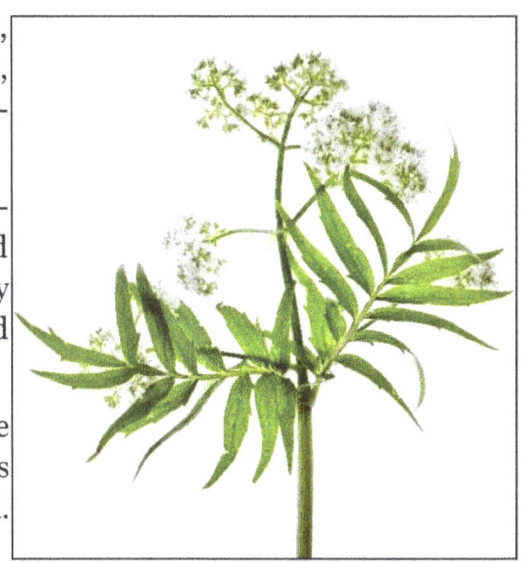

This includes pain from headaches, fibromyalgia, and nerve-related back issues. Make a strong tincture with the chopped roots by filling a sterile glass jar with the roots and completely covering them in at least 80 proof alcohol. Let this sit and infuse for four to six weeks before straining it out.

Take five to ten milliliters of this tincture under the tongue every four to six hours as needed for pain. Valerian root makes many people drowsy and is often used as a natural sleep-aid. Make sure you do not take it while operating heavy machinery.

3. Toothache Plant, *Acmella oleracea*

Toothache plant can be a godsend when you are struggling with mouth pain. This plant has the unique and somewhat surprising ability to completely numb the mouth when a bud is applied to the area where you are experiencing pain from a cavity or similar issue.

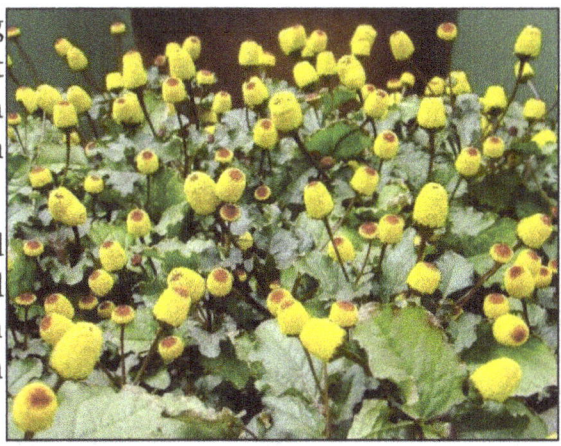

While a strong numbing effect can be felt with just one bud chewed in the mouth, you can harvest the buds and tincture them to create a numbing treatment to have on hand when you need it. To do this, simply fill a jar with toothache plant buds.

To create a strong tincture, try macerating the buds in a little 80 proof alcohol in a blender and then pouring this into the jar. Then top it off with more alcohol so that you have the plant material completely covered. Let this sit for four to six weeks before straining it out. To use, place a few drops in the mouth where you are experiencing pain and let them sit on the area as long as possible. You will begin to feel the numbing effects almost immediately. Apply a few drops as needed for pain.

4. Ginger

Ginger is known for its anti-inflammatory actions, but right along with the reduction in inflammation comes a reduction of pain when using this plant. Ginger has also been shown to increase blood circulation, helping to aid in healing to any areas where you may be experiencing pain. Many people swear by ginger for helping with migraines and headaches. It has also been used with success by those suffering from arthritis and

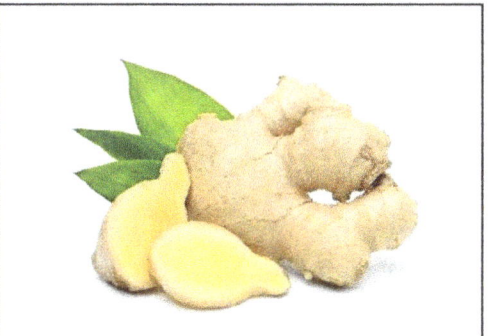

painful joints. You can drink ginger in tea, but to get a stronger formulation you should make a tincture with this plant. Start by finely chopping the root and filling a jar. Completely cover the chopped ginger in 80 proof alcohol and let this infuse for four-six weeks. Strain this out and add it in a dropper bottle. Take two-three droppers full every two hours as needed for pain.

5. White Willow, *Salix alba*

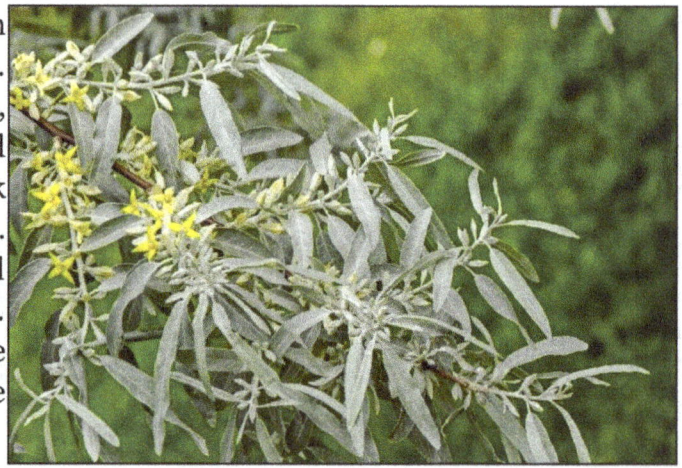

The beautiful white willow tree is where early man figured out how to cure pain using the inner bark. After centuries of utilizing this tree for pain, pharmaceutical companies caught on to this and discovered that the compound in the bark responsible for relieving pain is called salicin. Salicin was then extracted from the plant material and used to make what we know today as Aspirin. However, you can make your own "aspirin" at home by collecting the inner bark shavings from this tree and making a tincture.

Fill a jar with shavings of the inner bark and then completely cover this in alcohol. Strain it out after four to six weeks and bottle it. For an even stronger tincture, use the strained tincture to cover more bark shavings in a jar and strain this out again after four weeks. You will have a doubly strong salicin extract. Take two droppers full every two hours as needed for pain. This will also help reduce a fever if needed.

2. Antibiotics

Perhaps one of the most crucial medicines we might need in a serious situation are antibiotics. The advent of antibiotics saved many lives, but unfortunately, after a century of their use we now have to deal with strains of "super germs" that are resistant to many antibiotics. This is because antibiotics have been largely overprescribed and germs adapt, just like everything else. There are plants that work much like antibiotics in the body and can help to cure many types of infections, including throat infections, wounds, and urinary tract infections. The plants below have proven to have powerful antibiotic attributes.

1. Usnea

Usnea is a type of lichen that can be found on dead tree limbs. It is often called "Old man's beard." It has been utilized for its ability to fight a broad spectrum of infections including strep throat and staph infections.

To fully utilize this lichen, harvest it and fill a jar with what you collect. Wash it out well first, as bugs like to hide in it. When you have your jar filled, cover it with at least 80 proof alcohol and let this infuse for four to six weeks. Strain out the liquid after the allotted time and bottle it. For strep, gargle five to ten milliliters for one minute before swallowing it. Repeat this every three hours until the infection is gone. For staph, apply the tincture to boils every few hours and cover this with a bandage. You can also take five milliliters internally to cleanse staph from your system.

2. Goldenseal, *Hydrastis Canadensis*

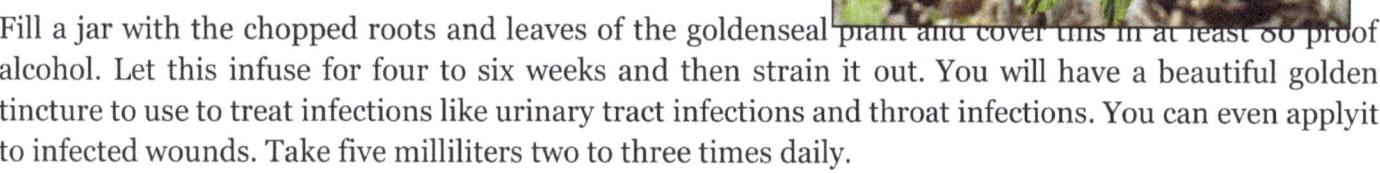

Goldenseal has been a highly sought-after plant for treating infections. So much so that it was overharvested for years in the Midwest. Now this plant has had a chance to flourish once again. The golden roots of this plant led to its name.

While the roots are powerful, when you tincture this plant, tincture the leaves as well. The leaves contain compounds that help make the healing properties in the roots more effective.

Fill a jar with the chopped roots and leaves of the goldenseal plant and cover this in at least 80 proof alcohol. Let this infuse for four to six weeks and then strain it out. You will have a beautiful golden tincture to use to treat infections like urinary tract infections and throat infections. You can even apply it to infected wounds. Take five milliliters two to three times daily.

3. Echinacea, *Echinacea* spp.

Echinacea is both antibiotic and antiviral. It helps the immune system fight various infections and viruses by giving it the boost it needs to fight off unwelcome guests. It makes an excellent companion with any of the other antibiotic herbs mentioned in this article to help tackle a variety of infections.

Create a tincture with the aerial parts of this plant and even a few chopped roots as well. Cover your plant parts in alcohol and let this infuse for four to six weeks. Strain it out and bottle the liquid. Try gargling five milliliters of Echinacea and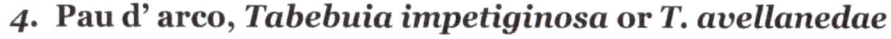
Usnea for a doubly powerful strep treatment. It also makes an excellent wound wash.

4. Pau d' arco, *Tabebuia impetiginosa* or *T. avellanedae*

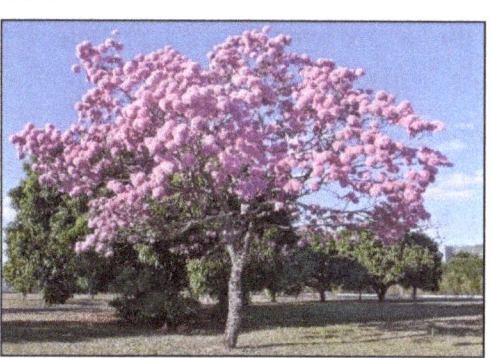

This powerful antibiotic treatment comes from the bark of a tree that grows in the rainforest. Pau d'arco is highly antibacterial and can help treat a variety of infections including urinary tract infections, throat infections, infected wounds, and more.

Create a strong decoction with the bark by adding four tablespoons of the bark to two cups of water in a pot on the stove. Let this boil until the liquid is reduced by half. Strain this out when it cools a bit and then use this to wash wounds, gargle for throat infections, or take internally. For internal use, take one half ounce every three hours. Refrigerate between uses and discard after two weeks.

5. Garlic, *Allium sativum*

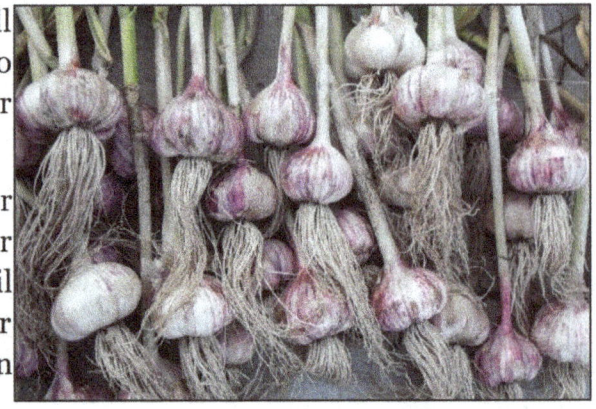

Garlic is one of the oldest remedies for infections and still remains one of the most powerful. One of the best ways to use garlic for infections is to infuse it in olive oil to treat ear infections.

Chop three cloves of garlic and add this to a double boiler with one cup of olive oil. Let this sit under low heat for eight hours and then strain it out. Let the olive oil infusion cool enough to comfortably drop inside the ear and lie on your side with this in your ear for ten to fifteen minutes. Repeat this with the other ear if necessary.

Garlic can also be taken internally for infections. You can treat bacterial vaginosis by inserting a garlic clove into the vagina for several hours each day or infusing several chopped cloves into coconut oil (similar to the recipe for the ear oil) and then straining this out to cool. When the coconut oil is almost fully solidified, roll it into a ball and insert it into the vagina at night before bed.

3. Anti-Inflammatories

Many pharmaceutical anti-inflammatories come at a price. This price is often damage to other organs and a dependence on using them often because their effects are very temporary. There are several anti-inflammatory plants that can help relieve inflammation, and as a result, pain and discomfort.

1. Cabbage, *Brassica oleracea*

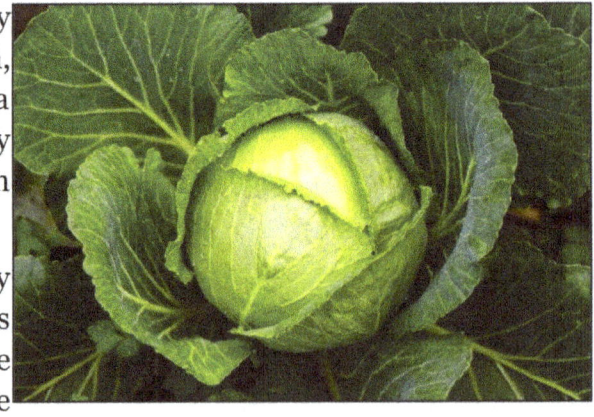

Cabbage leaves are one of the best anti-inflammatory treatments and they are so easy to come by! To use them, simply apply the leaf to the inflamed area, such as a sprained ankle. To maximize their effectiveness, apply plastic wrap over the cabbage leaves to hold them in place. You can reapply every few hours as needed.

Cabbage leaves also make an extremely effective remedy for the inflammation that comes with engorged breasts and mastitis. Simply apply the cabbage leaves to the breasts and you will notice an almost immediate reduction in swelling, fever, and pain.

2. Turmeric/ Curcumin

Turmeric is a close relative to ginger, so it's no surprise it works for inflammation and pain. Turmeric contains a compound called curcumin that helps to reduce inflammation and swelling in many areas of the body. It is great for back inflammation, chronic inflammation, autoimmune-related inflammation. Create a strong extract by chopping the roots and filling a jar. Completely cover the chopped roots in at least 80 proof alcohol and let this infuse for four to six weeks before straining it out. Take two to three droppers full up to three times a day to counter inflammation.

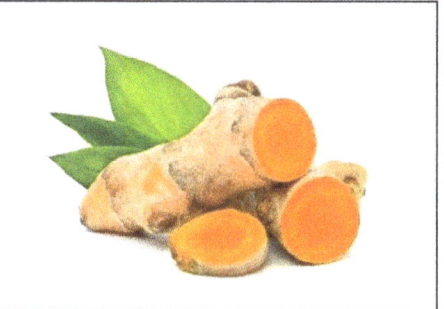

3. Black Pepper

Like turmeric, black pepper also contains anti-inflammatory compounds. In fact, it is recommended that you combine turmeric and black pepper for the best of both worlds and even better absorption into the body! To do this, when you fill your jar with chopped turmeric to make turmeric tincture, add two to three tablespoons of black pepper seeds. Follow the same protocol outlined above and strain it out after four to six weeks. Take two to three droppers full up to three times daily.

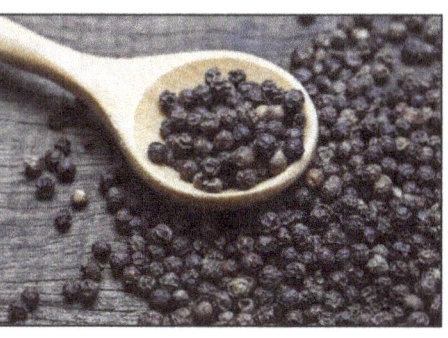

4. Aloe

Known for soothing external burns, Aloe also has powerful anti-inflammatory properties. One of the best ways to utilize it is to take it internally. It helps alleviate inflammation in the bowels caused by irritable bowel disease and similar maladies. It also helps to calm an inflamed urinary tract and bladder if you suffer from constant urinary tract infections or Interstitial Cystitis. Harvest the inner gel by slicing the leaves open and scraping it out. Bottle what you collect and add one to two ounces to smoothies. Drink one to two ounces daily. Only take enough to use each day or you will need to refrigerate the leftovers.

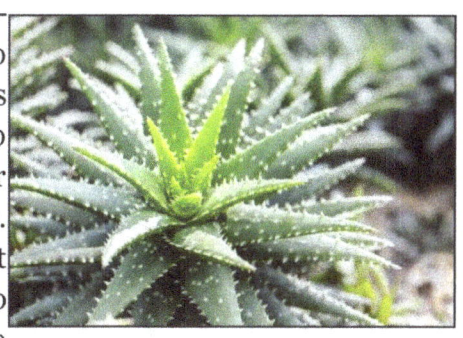

5. Goldenrod, *Solidago* spp.

Goldenrod is a powerhouse of antioxidant action, helping to significantly calm inflammation as well. If you suffer from inflammation in the stomach lining, bowels, bladder, or urinary tract, you may benefit from drinking one to two cups of golden rod tea as needed. Harvest the aerial parts in the fall and chop them finely. Add this to a tea infusion bag or tool and infuse this in a cup of hot water for ten minutes before consuming.

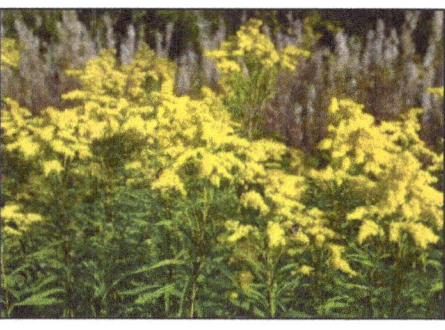

The plant world is full of surprises, but knowing that there are many options if you run out of vital pharmaceutical resources is one of the most pleasant surprises. Additionally, the fact that these plants have been used for centuries and have proven to provide gentle yet effective treatment is valuable.

www.ingramcontent.com/pod-product-compliance
Lightning Source LLC
Chambersburg PA
CBHW082249220526
45469CB00009B/2930